A Sociology of Family Life

Change and Diversity in Intimate Relations

DEBORAH CHAMBERS

polity

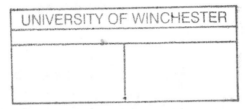

A Sociology of Family
Life

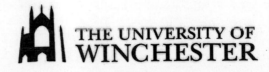

Contents

✦

Acknowledgements

I am grateful to Olwyn Ince for research assistance which helped the book progress to completion. I would also like to thank my colleagues in Humanities and Social Sciences at Newcastle University who have created a stimulating research culture from which I have benefited immeasurably, including events such as the Sociology Seminar Series and the Household Research Network (HoRNet) and various ESRC seminar series. In particular I'd like to mention David Baines, Richard Collier, Cathrine Degnen, Chris Haywood, Robert Hollands, Peter Hopkins, Helen Jarvis, Tracey Jensen, Stephanie Lawler, Janis McLaughlin, Daniel McNeil, Monica Moreno Figueroa, Anoop Nayak, Geoff Payne, Carolyn Pedwell, Peter Phillimore, Liviu Popoviciu, John Richardson and Yvette Taylor.

I am thankful for being invited to participate at events that have directly or indirectly helped develop and improve the book: the research forum on 'New Perspectives on Families, Intimacies and Care', Manchester Metropolitan University, 2010; the Ageing and Femininity series at the Center for the Study of the Americas (C. SAS), Karl-Franzens-University, 2010; and the 'Points of Exit: (Un)conventional Representations of Age, Parenting, and Sexuality' conference at the Centre for Gender and Diversity, Maastricht University, 2009. I am grateful to Emma Longstaff and Jonathan Skerrett at Polity Press for excellent guidance and support. My special thanks go to Lis Joyce for her moral support and encouragement.

Introduction

Recent scholarship on personal relationships and family life suggests that new kinds of love and commitment are being forged in contemporary societies. Relationships and living arrangements which are now commonplace include cohabiting couples, single-parent families, post divorce and 'blended' families, same-sex unions, 'friends as family', 'living apart but together' (LATS); and 'families of choice'. Family diversity has coincided with aspirations towards more 'democratic relationships'. The strong desire for more equal, more open and more egalitarian intimate relationships influences not only couples but also the way that parents relate to their children, with a new emphasis on childhood agency.

Rising divorce rates, teenage pregnancies, single parenthood, same-sex unions and cohabitation are often viewed as threats to the core of society. However, this book explains that these trends do not amount to evidence of a decline of commitment or responsibility for kin. The wide range of personal relationships and living arrangements in today's society is a sign that the concept of 'family' is becoming more fluid and changeable. The popularity of the term 'family', which is even being extended to describe close friendships and alternative kinds of intimacies, suggests a strong social desire to preserve principles of commitment and reciprocity that bind members of society together. This diversity in living arrangements thrives despite government attempts to *standardize* families through housing policies, tax breaks for married couples, divorce and post-divorce parenting laws, family planning, types of access to new reproductive technologies and so on. A principal objective of this book, then, is to document and analyse the growing variations in personal and family life and assess contemporary modes of commitment.

The increasing public recognition of family diversity has triggered alarm among certain politicians, religious leaders, academics and journalists. The welfare of children and elderly relatives is viewed as a major issue in an era of high divorce rates and rising single parenthood. Complex forms of commitment and care are being experienced by parents and wider kin at a time when governments in many countries are reducing social welfare provisions. A great deal of public debate about 'good' and 'bad' parenting has been fuelled by anxieties about a collapse of moral standards caused by the deterioration of 'proper' family values. Moral panics about 'family decline' expressed by governments and the media are regularly accompanied by calls to return to the apparently superior values of a past golden age of family life. Thus, although it is just one of many diverse living arrangements, the nuclear family remains a powerful icon of tradition and stability, often still perceived as an antidote to today's social problems.

The increase in family diversity – and negative responses to this trend from governments, academics and public bodies who promote a nuclear family norm – therefore comprises a key theme of this book. A second major theme is the study of families through a global lens. A range of transnational topics are dealt with across the chapters and examined in depth within a group of three key chapters. These three chapters focus on family migration and the globalization of intimate relations (chapter 6); the impact of population policies on fertility patterns (chapter 7); and the use of new reproductive technologies to create the 'perfect' or 'proper' family (chapter 8). The global themes are approached with a particular emphasis on family structures and relations in developing and under-developed countries. They look at how family life has been influenced by global labour migration, state policies and cultural values affecting fertility, arranged marriages and marriage migration.

The case-study examples drawn on from non-western societies are chosen according to the accessibility of reliable research data. The aim is to illustrate family customs, structures and patterns of social change that contrast with or challenge western assumptions about 'the family'. Reflecting the availability and relevance of research from these regions, a particular focus on India and China provides consistent threads. This is particularly the case in the chapters that deal with transnational family processes at a macro-sociological level by assessing how families negotiate wider and large-scale social systems including the link between globalization and marriage strategies, the regulation of families through state policies on population and fertility control, and transnational comparisons of the management and uses of reproductive technologies. All of these topics draw attention to the ways that state policies, religious and cultural customs and patriarchal structures regulate families and intimacies and are negotiated by individuals and families.

Themes and issues

In addition to the foregrounding of diversity and global dimensions of changing intimacies and family life, this book is arranged around a sequence of interrelated issues. The following broad questions frame these issues:

1. Is there sufficient research evidence to support the influential idea of a 'democratization' of family and intimate relationships, or are gender inequalities persisting in this context?
2. Is a growing diversity in intimate relationships leading to a crisis of commitment and care in western societies?
3. Is research on same-sex intimacies forcing a reconsideration of the concept of 'family'?
4. Are sociological debates about family life ethnocentric?

These questions are introduced in turn, below, and form key threads through the following chapters. They represent some of the major challenges associated with discrepancies between abstract social *theories* and empirical research *evidence* about family life.

With regard to the first question, the study of family life has recently been influenced by a refocus on the concept of 'intimacy', prompted by Anthony Giddens' book *The Transformation of Intimacy* (1992). His approach has stimulated extensive sociological debate. Giddens claims that changes in intimacy and family relationships in late twentieth-century western societies have led to a *democratization* of interpersonal relationships. He argues that sex has been separated from reproduction in late modernity. This is part of a trend of more equal and evenly balanced intimate interaction between couples which is said to be part of a liberalization of attitudes in western societies. This pattern corresponds with a stronger emphasis on individual self-fulfilment in personal relationships which, in turn, is part of a process of *individualization*.

Couples no longer feel bound by duty to get married before they have sex. They can decide these steps between themselves, as active agents, if and when they agree to. Giddens argues that this frees up the opportunity for a 'pure relationship' between the couple, a relationship in which men and women become equals. Individuals now expect much more from intimate relationships and are much more prepared to get divorced or move on to the next relationship if either party feels trapped or no longer feels fulfilled. Giddens argues that expectations of a life-long conjugal relationship involving having and bringing up children, with wife as homemaker and husband as breadwinner, have gone. Today, then, intimate relationships in western societies are more likely to be egalitarian and fluid, more temporary and short-lived and yet also more intense. He refers to this trend as a *detraditionalization* of intimacy.

These influential concepts of *individualization* and *detraditionalization* were advanced by 'late modern' social theory in the 1990s to explain changes in social and personal relationships. This perspective is also held by Ulrich Beck and Elizabeth Beck-Gernsheim (1995), as outlined in chapter 2. The current period of 'late modernity' is distinguished from an earlier period of 'modernity', up to around the mid twentieth century. Late modernity is viewed as a later phase of modernity rather than a break from it, in the sense of 'postmodern society'. These changes are important because they describe the changing condition of western societies in which tradition and social hierarchy are being questioned. Late modern social theorists argue that extended kinship ties and tight communities are being replaced by looser and more fragmented social ties. These wider social changes are said to have had dramatic effects on personal and family life.

More recent ways of approaching intimacy and sexuality in contemporary family relationships have been advanced by authors such as Lynn Jamieson (1998) and Neil Gross (2005). These authors represent a group of British and American academics who have engaged critically with the idea of *individualization*. Jamieson and Gross question the emphasis of the 'pure relationship' on self-obsessed individualism. The idea of the 'pure relationship' undermines the significance of everyday commitments and caring roles that make up family life, especially in parent–child relationships. A recurring theme of research findings outlined in the following chapters is the strength and durability of family and intimate ties. While personal relationships are clearly changing and adjusting to rising expectations of equality and intimacy in relationships, a compelling body of evidence indicates that commitment and reciprocity remain remarkably buoyant in terms of care for children and older relatives.

Turning to the second question, Jamieson also queries the idea that today's intimate relationships are now more equal, in the context of parental care for children. Discussions about 'parenting' often obscure the highly gendered practice of caring for children. Most of the caring work in and beyond families is still placed on women's shoulders. This issue is explored in depth in chapter 3 on parenting. Jamieson emphasizes that intimate relationships between men and women, and between children and parents, tend to be *asymmetrical* relationships structured by gender and generational relations of power. Thus, while addressing contemporary changes in intimacy and family relations, authors such as Jamieson have drawn attention to inequalities of gender and age that remain in family relationships. A further key theme that characterizes this book is, then, the continuing reproduction of unequal gender relations that shape families despite assertions of a 'democratization' of intimate relationships. Changes in parenting values and practices have coincided with women's rising educational levels and employment, control of fertility, divorce, changing employment patterns for men, and the decline of the 'breadwinner' ideal of the husband as the sole earner (see chapter 3).

Debates about parenting practices and values indicate that mothers tend to take responsibility for the day-to-day caring for children, despite attempts by governments to encourage fathers to become more involved in family life (Gillies 2005). In countries such as the USA and UK, the continuing imbalance in gender relations in the home is exacerbated by lack of childcare facilities for working parents. Women are still expected to sacrifice employment prospects for children rather than sharing the responsibilities with male partners. The following chapters confirm that governments continue to have a substantial impact on the size and structure of families. Yet the decline of welfare support for families in many countries with ageing populations is placing increasing pressures on women with families.

Referring to the third question about same-sex intimacies, significant advances in new scholarship have allowed the fixed categories of 'family' and 'parenting' to be contested or altered to suit changing intimacies. Research on gay, lesbian, bisexual and transsexual intimacies and queer theory have provided a critical reinterpretation of intimacy and personal life in recognition of the variability and

ͱes of today's family practices and personal lives. Following
ᵉrtain researchers argue that same-sex couples are more
ᵤhieve equality in their relationships. Since they are no
longer dependent on traditional gender roles, same-sex couples have
the opportunity to reinvent the ground rules in their daily lives in
areas such as performing household tasks (Weeks et al. 1999a and
1999b; see chapter 2). Through the use of donor reproductive technologies and surrogacy, same-sex couples are able to have children and
bring new approaches to parenting and household arrangements.
Rather than advancing a narrow idea of families as only functions of
the reproduction or socialization of children, contemporary sociology
highlights these major changes in intimacy and their implications
for changing family practices and conceptualizations of personal ties.

With regard to the final question, the lack of accurate historical
sociological data about minority ethnic kinship relations in western
societies is indicated in chapters that examine both macro- and
micro-social dynamics of family life. Past sociological research on
minority ethnic families has been characterized by an *ethnocentric*
bias: the predisposition for western academics to interpret minority
ethnic families from their own ethnic viewpoint. This bias has led to
a privileging of white and typically middle-class family norms and a
tendency to view that social unit as superior. Scholars, governments
and popular cultural discourses have been inclined to reify or natural-
ize the white nuclear family, even though it has only ever existed as
just one type of family among many others. The nuclear family is an
abstract ideal often treated as if it were a real and tangible object. As
an ideological construct it is elevated as a norm through a range of
official and informal discourses. The chapters of this book address
the ideological assumptions and misconceptions that contributed
to earlier and more recent sociological theory and policy debates
about 'the family'. These assertions are examined in relation to
empirical research evidence of actual families and people's lives in
order to identify and understand the richness and complexities of
contemporary familial and intimate relations.

Organization of the book

The book's chapters are organized in two broad ways. The first
comprises an outline of major theoretical perspectives followed by
critiques and reconsiderations generated by empirical studies. This

approach is used in chapters that deal with theories and debates about intimacy, parenting and childhood. For example, new scholarship on same-sex intimacies, parenting and household practices that contest apparently entrenched categories of 'family' and of parenting have redefined family practices. Examples of this body of research are then assessed to show how debates about family life and intimacy have been advanced. Likewise, scholarship on minority ethnic families and intimacies have either informed or challenged conventional thinking about family life, and are addressed to allow students to consider the discrepancies between standard and new ways of thinking about families. A second group of chapters are organized around a case-study approach. This approach is used in sections that address global themes including migration and marriage strategies, fertility and populations, and reproductive technologies. These sections draw on circumstances and events in specific countries through a comparative set of examples to illustrate key processes and changes in family forms and practices.

Chapter 1 traces the historical roots of key concepts of kinship and family in sociology. Foundational approaches to the family and kinship that developed in anthropology and sociology from the late nineteenth century to the 1980s are outlined. The way classical social theories defined family life and how their perspectives influenced modern thought are assessed. The roots of some of today's enduring ideas about 'the family' are uncovered by examining the perspectives of nineteenth-century thinkers such as Marx and Engels. The early twentieth-century structural-functionalist approach led by American sociologist Talcott Parsons proposed that the small, nuclear version of the family was perfectly adapted to the needs of modern society. He introduced new ideas about how the nuclear family's sex roles operate to reproduce the population and a stable workforce. The functionalist model has had a major impact on official discourses in the UK and USA about the ideal nuclear family. Chapter 1 also assesses the negative effects of functionalist approaches in studies of minority ethnic families in the USA and UK, in which extended and one-parent families were viewed as deviations from a nuclear family form.

Public and academic anxieties about loosening family ties in modern industrial societies proved to be unfounded, according to a range of empirical studies in the mid twentieth century. Informal relationships were shown to be highly significant at personal and structural levels. The principal feminist perspectives of the 1970s and

1980s on the family, sex, gender and patriarchy, which critiqued the functionalist perspective, are also addressed in chapter 1. Feminist models revealed the ways in which the institution of 'the family' reproduces patriarchal, heterosexual versions of masculinity and femininity. Feminist perspectives contributed to an understanding of how inequalities of gender, class and race are reproduced through family and wider social structures and relations.

Public concerns about the erosion of mutual responsibility and long-term commitment lie at the heart of arguments about a decline in family values. In chapter 2, theories and debates from the 1990s about changes in intimate relationships are examined. The use of the concept of 'individualization' to explain the rise of more egalitarian intimate relationships is assessed in depth. The chapter explains, in detail, changing ideas about love and commitment, the altering nature of the self and society and the rise of the 'pure relationship'. These explanations are queried through a range of empirical research which is addressed in the second half of the chapter. A series of recent and mainly qualitative research on intimacy has provoked a reassessment of late modern theory and fed into critiques of the individualization thesis.

Debates about changes in parenting values and practices are assessed in chapter 3. Changing notions and practices of motherhood, highlighted by feminist debates, have corresponded with women's improved education and entrance into the labour market. The identification of a 'new' parenthood that emerges out of separation and divorce has affected definitions and practice of both mothering and fathering (Smart 1999). The rise of lone parenting, teenage parents, post-divorce families and parenting within minority ethnic families are addressed. This is followed by a focus on current ideas about fatherhood. New models of fatherhood have been prompted by the erosion of the male breadwinner role, the rise in post-divorce families and families absent of fathers. Public discourses on a new kind of Dad based on the model of 'involved' or 'active fatherhood' are displacing the notion of the father as 'male breadwinner' and unemotional disciplinarian. Fatherhood is being reconstructed in law and social policy, a theme explored against the backdrop of changing modes of heterosexual masculinity and changing patterns of male employment (Smart and Neale 1999; Collier 1999; Collier and Sheldon 2008). The idea of 'involved fatherhood' being promoted by the state in the UK and USA is addressed. The chapter looks at research evidence about how estranged couples cope with bringing up children after divorce. The parenting patterns of minority ethnic families are also examined as important factors in the construction of new parenting practices. In the final section, changing ideas about parenting advanced by gay, lesbian and bisexual parents are discussed, including the recent struggles that members of the gay and lesbian community have experienced in defending the right to parent.

Chapter 4 traces changes in the nature of childhood. It highlights the tensions between opposing accounts of childhood: a traditional romantic ideal which affirms the right of a child to be innocent and protected and the idea of the child as an active agent with rights. The practicalities of contemporary childrearing practices are set against this romantic ideal and can lead to confusion for both parents and children. Childrearing is now depicted as a negotiation between parent and child, within a process monitored by the state and other agencies such as schools. The impact of post-divorce families, lone parenting and poverty on childhood are examined. Contemporary approaches to childhood draw attention to children's accelerating contact with the media, commercialism and new technologies. This exposure has complicated the idealized and sentimental notion of childhood. The chapter also shows that in certain parts of the non-western world, childhood is being shaped by elements of privatized and individualized family life familiar to western societies. This suggests that a western trend of home-based, privatized childhoods may be a globalizing tendency. Changes taking place in contemporary urban China are outlined to offer an insight into the way these changes are impacting transnationally.

Chapter 5 on families and ageing societies identifies the key ways in which family relationships are being transformed within the life course. The term 'life course' is used in sociology to indicate an individual's passage through life and is generally studied as a sequence of significant life events that include birth, marriage, parenthood, divorce and retirement. It replaces the traditional term 'life-cycle' which contained too many normative implications about the 'correct' sequencing of the stages that people go through. Major changes in family responsibilities over the life course have been driven by increases in life expectancy, an extension of the age of reproduction and longer periods of 'post-parental' life, as well as rising divorce rates. Patterns of reciprocity between older and younger family members show that older relatives, particularly women, often take on significant responsibilities as grandparents. The chapter looks at ageing and intergenerational ties and examines how families and households deal with the anxieties of caring for the elderly in western and in developing societies. Various configurations of social support, including friends, neighbours and extended kin, are now involved in caring in an ageing society. This is particularly the case among non-traditional family forms, such as gay, lesbian and bisexual couples. New research agendas prompted by the globalization of family life are being developed, in which the preservation of generational and network-based ties across different nation states are being documented and analysed (Levitt 2001; Phillipson et al. 2006). The chapter therefore also addresses the impact of migration on the care of the elderly.

Scholars have tended to study globalization in terms of capital, state and market mechanisms, and new technologies (Harvey 1989; Johnson et al. 2002). In chapter 6, globalization is approached in a different manner. The ways that families negotiate and are affected by international migration and other transnational connections are addressed. How patterns of marriage and global processes have strengthened, reshaped or destabilized families is analysed. Local family systems and relations interconnect with and support large-scale processes of economic globalization through local practices and customs of kinship and marriage. The chapter is divided into two sections. The first section examines the growing mobility and global migration of families or family members, generated by the demand for care workers in the West. It raises important questions about the global political economy of formal and informal care. The second section examines transnational marriage strategies that form part of geographical and social mobility. Academic responses to transnational marriage are often influenced by western values of romance, such as the idea of the 'pure relationship'. These values imply that commercial imperatives in spouse selection undermine the authenticity of the marital relationship. Transnational marriage is often viewed as a business deal that transforms a kinship association into a form of human 'trafficking' (Palriwala and Uberoi 2008). The chapter examines the ways that marriage is exploited for social and economic mobility, including arranged marriages and commercially negotiated marriage, 'mail-order brides' and internet dating.

The theme of families and fertility is examined in chapter 7 through a series of historical and contemporary case studies that have gained currency in global debates about population and fertility control. National population issues including birth control, family planning, infant mortality and unsafe abortions are investigated. How religious and cultural customs, state policies and global agencies have addressed fertility and influenced family structures and values transnationally is explored. A dramatic shift in the field of population and development was prompted in 1994 by the International Conference on Population and Development. The ICPD produced a programme of action which recognized that reproductive health and rights, women's empowerment and gender equality should underpin all population and development programmes. This was triggered by several issues including revelations about the extent of misery inflicted on families by the population policies of Romania under the brutal dictatorship of Ceausescu between 1966 and 1989. The state and traditional customs in western and non-western cultures coalesced in regulating fertility and family practices. The aggressive family and demographic policies of the Ceausescu regime are described as a case study to demonstrate how women were coerced by the state into bearing children (Kligman 1998).

The second and third case studies addressed in this chapter involve the impact of son preference and modern population policies on families, in particular on the lives of women and children. Son preference is a deep-rooted cultural norm in Third World countries. How this custom has been defended and negotiated in relation to government attempts at fertility control and the availability of sex-selective abortion technologies is described in the context of India's family planning policies and China's 'one-child' policy. The cases are chosen because they occur in two of the most highly populated countries of the world with some of the most highly controversial and problematic sets of practices and customs. As such, they raise a number of key issues about the relationship between state policy and cultural traditions in the formation of family life.

Son preference and family sex composition are powerful customs that place pressure on women to make fertility decisions which conform to a deeply held tradition about the composition of the 'proper family'. Sex-selective abortions in India have skewed the ratio of boys to girls. The impact of this practice on the lives of women and girls, and government attempts to curtail the practice, are examined. How China's family planning programme, known as the 'one-child' policy, has changed fertility preferences forms the third case study. The effectiveness of this dramatic population policy is linked to its unique system of government control. The strong tradition of son preference in existence in China for more than 2,000 years continues to be a factor discouraging compliance with the policy. 'Demographic transition' in developed regions such as Europe and Japan, where the birth rates are lower than the death rate, is also addressed in this chapter to illustrate the ways governments attempt to increase family size and address ageing societies.

By exploring another way in which government policies impact on families' fertility decisions, chapter 8 addresses the effects of new reproductive technologies in a number of societies and among particular ethnic groups. The chapter summarizes controversies about the moral dilemmas surrounding in-vitro fertilization (IVF), assisted reproduction and surrogate motherhood. The legal regulation and restrictions imposed on the use of these technologies highlight the complexities involved in definitions of parenthood and often expose the ideology that binds ideas about kin. Issues of legitimacy are called into question by reproductive technologies. Where motherhood and fatherhood were once inevitable and given, they now require definition by law. Ethnic and religious differences, migration and the effects of globalization are examined. Discrepancies between government policy and family fertility practices in the Middle East and India are addressed. Feminist debates are drawn on and assessed to illustrate the role they play in understanding these past and present practices.

The final chapter addresses three key themes that characterize the book as a whole, to demonstrate the major challenges that have faced sociological developments in the study of family and intimate life. The first is the prominence of sociological theories that perceive a decline in commitment and trust in family and intimate relations. Traditional family values are evoked by governments to identify and defend the moral standards of the nation (Stacey 1999). This family values discourse is regularly expressed in the political speeches of heads of state. Politicians are aware that a discourse of family crisis and the promotion of a nuclear family form is a vote catcher. This ideology is addressed in the final chapter since it sets the parameters of public debate and has serious implications for policy formation and scholarship on family and personal life.

The second section foregrounds key ways in which the biological idea of family relations is being challenged and reconfigured. It addresses concepts which are inclusive and flexible enough to address newer relationships beyond conventional nuclear or heterosexual family forms, such as same-sex relationships, cohabitation, friendships, single-parent families, post-divorce unions and reconfigured kinship networks. For example, Carol Smart advances the term 'personal life' to explain the significance of personal connectedness and the embeddedness of relations. The third section also highlights major ways in which non-kin relations are taking on family-like meanings and being included in the study of intimacy and family life. Other kinds of intimacy such as friendship are also drawn on to describe 'family' or 'family-like' relationships. 'Friend-like relationships' and the voluntary nature of relationships are now increasingly being privileged over compulsory relationships bound by duty. Yet these friend-like relationship types are enhancing kin ties rather than replacing them. Spencer and Pahl (2006) develop the concept of 'personal communities' to describe new kinds of relationships evolving in late modernity. They contradict public and political fears that social bonds are being weakened and leading to a breakdown of family and social cohesion. The fourth section details the lead taken by queer theory in addressing and celebrating the new kinds of intimacies and household arrangements that draw on the concept of friendship and community to authenticate relationships that were once stigmatized and rendered marginal.

The final section highlights the importance of examining the interconnection between intimacy and global processes. The section addresses sociological reassessments of the traditional, false separation of 'public' and 'private' spheres of society by drawing attention to the relationship between economic and intimate spheres of life. It calls for a fusion of macro- and micro-sociological methods and debates to advance our understanding of the ways in which public and private realms of politics and work correspond with intimacy and family. The chapter illustrates this by addressing the affective economic analyses of Arlie Hochschild (2003b) and Viviana Zelizer (2005) to highlight the ways that family and intimate life are shaped by and influence economic exchanges. This is obvious in cases such as commercial marriage transactions and commercial surrogacy but less so in emotional and caring practices. This body of work highlights the connection between economic, emotional and caring practices in family relationships.

1 Traditional Approaches to the Family

Sociological accounts of family and personal relationships in the nineteenth and early twentieth centuries were characterized by anxieties about the decline of traditional family values. This perception of 'family decline' has persisted to the present day, forming part of a broader set of concerns about the break-up of community ties. Rising *individualism* and *privatization* were identified among the causes. It was argued that neighbours no longer supported or knew one other; families became more insular; traditional forms of respect and deference were weakening; and individuals were becoming more self-absorbed and materialistic. By the mid twentieth century, these fears of moral decline coincided with anxieties about the break-up of the nuclear family. It was feared that rising individualism would lead to an abandonment of marriage, particularly by women. The idea of the 'companionate marriage' was introduced to address the dilemma.

This chapter outlines key approaches to family and kinship studies from the late nineteenth to the twentieth century that prompted these kinds of anxieties about family decline. The first sections look at late nineteenth-century perspectives that aimed to prove or disprove the universality of a particular kind of family. These sections outline late nineteenth-century anthropological influences on early sociological debates in America and Britain, and address the contrasting socialist study of the family by Frederick Engels which highlighted women's status in relation to production, reproduction and capitalism. The second part of the chapter addresses moral anxieties about a decline of family values associated with the dominant approaches to the family in the early and mid twentieth century. Most twentieth-century theories about the family examined the effects of the process of industrialization and urbanization on family structures. For example, the influential structural-functionalist perspective represented by American sociologist Talcott Parsons approached the modern nuclear family as a unit shaped by the needs of capitalism. The family transformed from a producing to a consuming unit.

The third section addresses studies that contradicted views of moral decline associated with a weakening of family ties. The classic British urban community studies of kinship of the 1950s and early 1960s show some of the ways that empirical research refuted sociological anxieties about family and community decline. In the fourth section, feminist debates of the 1970s and 1980s are outlined to introduce new critiques of certain assumptions in earlier sociological work. Feminist scholars drew attention to gendered relations of power in both the domestic and public spheres of society. They exposed the ideological nature of gendered power relations and how they placed structural constraints on women in the family and in other areas of society, including restricted and low-paid employment for women. Chapter 2 builds on these themes and issues by assessing more recent social theories from the 1990s that have come to dominate contemporary sociological debates about changes in gender relations, sexual identities and family structures and meanings. In this chapter, we move from the nineteenth- to the mid- twentieth-century themes and issues.

Late nineteenth-century sociological perspectives

Many early sociological ideas about marriage, the family and kinship in the late nineteenth century were influenced by the related discipline of anthropology. During this period, anthropology was preoccupied with biological discourses of relatedness. The institution of marriage was traditionally viewed as biologically determined to address three needs: procreation and the rearing of children; the lengthy period of dependence of children on their parents; and the need for prolonged parental care and training. Through biological relatedness, individuals recognized as kin were divided into those related by blood (consanguines) and those related by marriage (affines). Clearly, biological blood ties dominate the ordering of social relations in societies where procreation is a defining characteristic of relatedness (Beattie 1964). However, contemporary studies of kinship now acknowledge that forms of family relatedness are also socially constructed, as in cases of adoption, same-sex unions including those with children, single-parent households, step-relations and also donor-assisted conception (see chapter 8). Nevertheless, even though biology is not the only basis of kinship, biological relatedness continues to have a powerful impact on ideas about the structuring of kin.

The social significance given to biological 'blood ties' as the defining features of 'family' can be illustrated in a variety of ways. Examples include DNA testing to prove biological parentage; the attempt made by adopted children to find their biological parents; and the current public fascination with family history. Television programmes and the publicity devoted to following adopted individuals who try to trace their 'real mother' show that genetic connection remains a paramount element of identity (Stanworth 1987). These practices indicate the fascination in western societies for discovering the 'self' through biological heritage. DNA testing has reunited slave descendants of Afro-Caribbean origin with populations in Africa and Equatorial Guinea, for example. Such attempts reveal the social, legal and symbolic significance of blood relations, at both societal and individual levels (Taylor 2005). How this family connection through blood is both promoted and complicated will be considered further in the context of new reproductive technologies in chapter 8.

Much traditional anthropological work on kinship and marriage in the nineteenth century was concerned not only with biological relatedness but also with classifying kin relationships in other cultures. Versions of these ties would then be selected to validate contemporary western family structures as universal, to confirm their naturalness. A bewildering variety of marriage types across the world were documented by anthropologists, including monogamy (having only one spouse), polygamy (having more than one wife or husband at a time) and polyandry (having more than one husband at a time); matriarchal (woman as ruler of the family) and patriarchal (man as ruler of the family) unions; households with matrilocal residence (move to the wife's home) and patrilocal residence (move to the husband's home). The aim of early sociological studies of the family was to navigate a path through these variations to create hypothetical constructions about 'original' or 'prior' forms of marriage. The aim was to *prove* that the acceptable version of monogamous marriage is the final, correct and highest stage of social evolution.

Given that kin relations in western societies were thought to have their roots in nature, analogies with the animal kingdom were often made by referring to the mating behaviour of higher primates. This allowed sociologists to bypass the awkward diversity of kinship types uncovered by early anthropology. Despite the lack of any existing representative examples, evolutionary schemes were devised from selected aspects of existing 'simple societies' to prove a natural earlier stage of marriage organization. For instance, the nineteenth-century evolutionary anthropologist Lewis Morgan constructed an evolutionary scheme in *Systems of Consanguinity and Affinity in the Human Family* (1870) in which he interpreted matriliny (descent through the female line) as preceding patriliny (descent through the male line) and monogamy as the final evolutionary stage.

Morgan's position was refuted by Edward Westermarck in his *History of Human Marriage* (1921), first published in 1891. He contested the hypothesis that primitive societies were promiscuous, believing that humans were originally monogamous. For proof, Westermarck used a biological discourse influenced by the ideas of Charles Darwin. He relied on selected examples of monogamy both among anthropoid apes and among hunter-gatherer peoples who were considered by social evolutionists as the most primitive societies. In this way, Westermarck argued that the nuclear family was prefigured among the anthropoids and was therefore the primary and universal unit from which contemporary society evolved. The child's need for parental protection generates the need for a family as a unit for the continued existence of certain species. The male remains with the female and child to *protect* them, and this is governed by instincts achieved through natural selection. These kinds of anthropological attempts at explaining kinship and marriage were no more than elaborate hypotheses. Yet they were accepted among the academic and wider communities because biological determinism supported a particular ideology to identify and reaffirm a 'proper' kind of family.

However, by the early twentieth century it became increasingly clear that bonds of family require *social recognition* rather than relying simply on the issue of *biological procreation*. Anthropologists were finding that, especially in societies beyond the so-called 'West', kinship is defined by *social* as well as *blood* ties. Societies were being discovered in which the physiological role of the male in reproduction was not recognized. In certain non-western societies, little or no significance is attached to the relationship between sexual union and the arrival of a baby nine months later. The husband regarded a child born to his wife as his own simply because she was his wife. In parts of Melanesia, for instance, it was found that the family to which a child belongs is not determined by the physiological act of birth but by the performance of some social act (Malinowski 1932).

In their book, *The Family: From Institution to Companionship* (1945), American sociologists Burgess and Locke defined the modern family as nuclear, describing it as a group of people united by marriage, blood or adoption. This family group was defined as constituting a single household whose members interacted with one another in their respective social roles of husband and wife, mother and father, brother and sister, to create a common culture. Importantly, then, Burgess and Locke included not only blood ties but also the *social* family tie of adoption in their definition of the modern family. However, this social family tie was underlined by the practical requirement that a man should publicly acknowledge himself to be a child's 'father'.

Engels: family, private property and the state

Many of the prominent political ideologies preceding the twentieth century failed to advance the cause of women. The idea that the position of women in society is an indicator of social progress emerged through the eighteenth-century Scottish Enlightenment. But this did not yet translate into equal rights for the sexes (Therborn 2004). Although science overtook religion as the established authority for advancing knowledge in the nineteenth century, gender inequality and women's inferiority persisted in scientific discourse. The rationale for gender difference was now established by Nature, rather than God. With his colleague Karl Marx, Frederick Engels challenged this account by arguing that women's oppression was treated as fixed and unchangeable. Engels explained religious or 'natural' accounts as flawed ideological rationalizations used to support a system of exploitation. He argued that the family was an unnatural institution designed to 'privatize' wealth and human relationships. Engels' book *The Origin of the Family, Private Property and the State* (1884) is a seminal work that traced the evolution of family organization from prehistory to the present. It comprised a historical approach to the family in relation to the issues of social class, female suppression and ownership of private property. His aim was to offer a social explanation for women's oppression with regard to the rise of the patriarchal family and private property at a particular historic period. This explanation was quite daring for the time because it challenged the dominant views that women's inferior status was God-ordained or founded on biological, physical, intellectual and moral inferiority.

According to Engels, the traditional monogamous family household was a recent concept that supported capitalist, property-owning societies. He argued that the division of labour and commodity exchange between individuals emerged as social class distinctions at this last phase of social evolution, and that the repression of women then became clearly visible. He explained that the patriarchal nature of the current family system was one in which women are not only servants to men but, to all intents and purposes, prostitutes. Engels claimed that liberation from class and gender oppression was possible for all. He argued that, in the beginning, people lived in unrestricted sexual intercourse which prevented a sure way of determining parentage. Descent could only be traced by the female line in compliance with matriarchal law and this was universally practised by nations of antiquity. As mothers, women received respect and deference which led to complete rule by women (gynaecocracy). The shift to monogamy, in which a certain woman was reserved exclusively to one man, undermined the primeval religious law of sexual freedom. For Engels, property and inheritance through family ties prevent people from engaging in free, passionate relationships. He argued that only through socialism could 'individual sex love' occur and that a Communist society could lead to communal living, equality, sexual freedom and the collapse of the state.

Engels has been criticized by feminist writers for not giving sufficient weight to feminist issues since he was more interested in economic production and capitalism than in the family and women. Although Engels distinguished between social production and reproduction, he subsumed reproduction under production because he claimed that women's liberation was dependent on economic liberation (Evans 2011). Engels' work has also been criticized for using inaccurate anthropological sources. Nevertheless, his book represented a significant critique of the Victorian nuclear family and continues to reverberate as a daring critique of sexual inequality. By studying the connection between patriarchy and capitalism, he was able to address the question of sexual inequality and the family, both *historically and politically*. By exploring how social divisions arise through the family, Engels identified both production and reproduction as the material bases of society. This approach has therefore been a key resource for subsequent sociologists in theorizing the intersection of class and gender structures. Engels made a significant contribution to feminist theory, sociology and methodology. However, in the early twentieth century, American sociological studies were more concerned with explaining a systematic connection between the structures of capitalism and the composition of the family.

The twentieth-century functional family

Sociologists of the twentieth century continued the focus on the relationship between the family unit and economic organization as a major theme. However, this was set against the backdrop of concerns about the idea of a loss of community and the impact on 'family'. For example, Ferdinand Tonnies (1955 [1887]) argued that, before the industrializing process, people lived in relatively small communities and therefore knew one another well, were highly interdependent and generated high levels of informal checks and controls on people. Later, with the rise of individual wage labour, these dependencies that bound the family together were weakened. Ties dependent on common property and inheritance among farming families were eroded with the rise of wage labour under industrialization.

Talcott Parsons, who outlined the basic principles of modern structural functionalism, viewed society as a social system defined in terms of 'needs' or 'functions'. For Parsons, the different parts of each society contribute positively to the operation or functioning of the system as a whole. In this respect, he regarded the institution of the nuclear family as functional for the operation of industrial society as a system. He argued that the extended family of pre-industrial society was no longer viable. The family was necessarily transformed by industrialization from an extended, economic unit of *production* in rural societies into a small, mobile nuclear unit of *consumption* in urban society (Parsons 1956; Parsons and Bales, 1956). Industrialization demands greater geographical and social mobility from its workforces. So the family unit shrank in size to adapt to this new economy. The large extended family of former times typically housed three generations of relatives under one roof, with several children and was characterized by wide but durable kinship ties. By contrast, the new, lean, nuclear family of the 1950s comprised two parents and two children who lived independently from grandparents or other relatives. During industrialization, functions once performed by the family, particularly production and education, were taken over by the state or outside institutions. Although the nuclear family lost certain functions, it became a more specialized institution that provides for socialization, emotional needs and mutual support of its members. Functions that the family provided in the way of care or financial support for extended kin became 'optional' functions since these services had been taken over in industrial societies by specialist institutions such as social services and hospitals.

By concentrating on reproducing the next generation, through the rearing and socialization of children, the nuclear family adapted efficiently to supply certain fundamental needs of modern society. So, for Parsons, the two key functions of the family were *primary socialization* and the *stabilization of adult personalities* (Parsons and Bales 1956). Primary socialization is the practice of teaching children the cultural norms and values of the society. The family was viewed by Parsons as the essential context for children's development of human personality. Personality stabilization concerns the role played by the family in supporting the emotional needs of adults as well as children. Parsons argued that healthy, stable adult personalities are maintained through marriage. In pre-industrial societies this stabilizing function was said to be performed by extended kin. An essential role of the family in industrialized society, then, was the creation of a stable context for the socialization of its members.

The nuclear family was viewed by Parsons as the most efficient unit for dealing with the challenges of modern society through a specialization of roles between husband and wife. This new kind of family relied on the allocation of 'instrumental' and 'affective' roles between husband and wife. The husband was expected to adopt the *instrumental role* of breadwinner and work outside the home while the wife was expected to adopt the *affective role* of attending to the emotional and domestic needs of the family. Men's instrumental role allowed them to adapt to paid employment outside the home. Women's expressive role was tailored to childcare and domestic work. Through these family roles, this intimate nuclear family was able to specialize in serving the emotional needs of adults and children to facilitate the adaptation of family members for a competitive and impersonal world beyond the home. Through family socialization, individuals acquired an understanding of how family relationships *should* behave and dutifully replicated this behaviour themselves. Within the framework of structural functionalism, then, these changes in family structure were explained by the needs of a capitalist economy. This new, smaller and more geographically mobile unit was viewed as *morally superior* and more efficient than that of the old extended family. Capitalism demanded small families as units of consumption capable of adjusting themselves to fit in with a new kind of employment market based on a particular gendered division of labour. The weakening of pre-industrial extended family ties was viewed as a progressive trend. It coincided with an erosion of traditional modes of nepotism in favour of meritocracy.

The functionalist explanation of change in family structures and roles was criticized by social historians and sociologists in a number of ways, and eventually discredited. First, the theory was criticized for advancing an abstract version of 'family' that relied on an abstract version of 'society' that required the reproduction of particular social forms. Second, it neglected the role played by other institutions outside the family in socializing children, such as government, education and the media. Third, functionalism was criticized by feminist scholars for naturalizing and justifying the unequal domestic division of labour between women and men. This 'modern functional family' legitimated the male 'breadwinner' model within an asymmetrical patriarchal structure. Fourth, functionalism privileged continuity to such an extent that social change was perceived negatively as a failure of the system. The approach was unable to explain many social problems in American society, including poverty, social conflict and class struggle. Finally, the approach neglected and was unable to explain family forms that deviated from the nuclear model. Research by anthropologists, historians and feminist scholars emphasizes the diversity of families not only across cultures and historical periods but also within cultures and periods. Functionalism ignored evidence of the persistence of extended kinship networks in certain locations and classes, and among certain non-white and ethnic minority groups (Macfarlane 1979; Davidoff et al. 1999; Laslett 2005 [1965]). The model was criticized for privileging a white, suburban and middle-class 'ideal'. Families that did not conform to this model were viewed as deviant.

Despite the theoretical deficiencies of functionalism, this perspective prevailed as the theoretical standard for most family sociology through to the 1970s. Indeed, mid-twentieth-century research on the 'modern family' and families of the past was framed by the functional model and therefore reinforced the idea that family structure naturally graduated from an extended to nuclear form. Selective research tended to refer to white families and western developments to confirm a particular pattern. An extensive re-examination of the question of a 'Golden Age' of the 1950s American family has since been prompted by a range of research that disputes earlier historical assumptions. The misleading conclusions of many earlier historical studies triggered an academic reconsideration about the notion of a past 'ideal family'. More recent historians discovered that family life was much more complex and diverse than previously assumed. For example, before the twentieth century, adoption of relatives' children was common; a high level of cohabitation without marriage occurred; and men often left former partners to form new intimate relationships and households with other women without supporting first wives and children (see, for example, Davidoff et al. 1999; Bailey 2003; Klein 2005). By the 1970s, feminist critiques were challenging many of the assumptions associated with the functional approach that had elevated a particular model of family as standard. However, since the functionalist approach was highly influential in its time, it had an enduring negative effect not only on the way that gender relations were studied but also on the ways that minority ethnic families and same-sex unions were researched, as addressed below.

Companionate marriage

Although Parsons argued that the modern nuclear family had adopted functions to support capitalism, this ideology generated anxiety among many sociologists. It was feared that the values of materialism and consumerism, associated with urban society, would contribute to a fragmentation of family life. Carle Zimmerman (1947) considered the urban American family of the 1940s and 1950s to be a disturbing sign of family disintegration. He argued that the family could no longer adequately carry out vital functions such as reproduction and socialization, stating that 'unless some unforeseen renaissance occurs, the family system will continue headlong its present trend towards nihilism' (1947:808). Burgess and Locke (1945) claimed that the model of the American family was transforming from an *institution* to a *companionship* in response to the disintegration of the traditional systems of control that had once stabilized the extended version of the family. Individuals expected more personal autonomy in their lives and fewer family restrictions. The loss of the economic function of families coincided with a stronger accent on the cultural purpose of families in fostering individual fulfilment. This shift was also linked with resettlement from sociable rural communities to more anonymous urban and suburban settings.

Burgess (1973) argued that, together with the rise of outside influences such as the media and popular culture, widespread social changes were causing family instability. Women were targeted as particular problems to society. They were becoming more self-seeking and individualistic through a loosening of patriarchal ties that had traditionally bound them to their families. Women's increasing independence endangered the permanence of the nuclear family, which was structured to address men's, not women's, personal needs. In response, the *companionate marriage* was an ideology deployed to defuse feminine individualism and evoke a new kind of egalitarian family (Finch and Summerfield 1991; Cheale 2002). The ideology of 'companionship' in marriage emerged, then, out of these concerns to forge an ideal of conjugal friendship. The aim was to protect the family against an invasion of selfish individualism. In the wake of traditional community decline and the rise of more alienated modes of urban living, the companionate marriage was treated as a kind of insurance: a necessary constituent of married life that glued heterosexual couples together.

This friendship marriage promoted the idea of an exclusive relationship that was to be mutually satisfying at an emotional and physical level for both partners. It evoked an egalitarian rapport between the spouses. Yet the ideal was bolted on to a traditional patriarchal model of the family, defined by a male head of household as the 'breadwinner' with a dependent female homemaker. This ideal was evoked in societies where women could not vote and had restricted access to both education and employment (Smart 2007). The apparently incompatible features of patriarchal power and control were combined with private, sexual and emotional dimensions of conjugal relationships. Nevertheless, public acceptance of the companionate marriage fostered the idea of a separation of reproduction from sexual pleasure. This elevation of sexual pleasure signified a fundamental shift in thinking because it promoted the belief that marriage was not simply a means to having children, even though this was still perceived as a key function of 'the family'. As David Cheale (1999) argues, the companionate marriage was an antidote to the encroaching values of individualism, but married couples could only make this transition with the help of experts. An army of family experts, such as sexologists, child guidance clinics, marriage counselling centres, psychiatrists and clinical psychologists, were at hand to sort out the problems of children and adults. A variety of 'therapeutic agencies' were established to prop up this new isolated, lonely nuclear family.

Community and kinship studies

Ideas about the decline of communal relations, the privatization of social life and a disintegration of family values continued to dominate academic and public debates of the 1950s and 1960s. Since industrialization, traditional commitments were being replaced by new kinds of loyalties and commonalities influenced by wider social and economic changes beyond the family, such as consumerism and geographical and social mobility. Changes in the structure of housing were also thought to be changing social ties. For example, after World War II, between the late 1940s and 1960s, the clearance of slum areas in Britain and other parts of war-torn Europe coincided with the building of new housing estates on the edge of urban areas which weakened traditional working-class communities (Crow and Allan 1994). Governments and academics feared that higher standards of new housing stock were accompanied by lower levels of social participation and less informal support so that families often felt isolated (Mogey 1956; Willmott and Young 1960; Willmott 1963; Crow and Allan 1994). Sociologists expressed concern about the decline of civic participation and the sense of atomization associated with isolated, individual nuclear families that become more inwardly focused on internal domestic matters.

Sociologists were also concerned with the problem of marriage breakdown and divorce, during the mid twentieth century. However, a series of classic kinship studies conducted in Britain during that period indicated that the notion of a 'decline' or 'death' of kinship had been overstated. Research documented changes in the context of modernity and uncovered the richness of family life, highlighting the strength of generational ties. For example, Young and Willmott's classic study of *Family and Kinship in East London* (1957, 1987) underlined the importance and positive value of extended family bonds despite widespread social changes, as did Townsend's *The Family Life of Old People* (1957). Kinship support was accepted as a normal aspect of everyday life and there was little evidence of segregated nuclear family units. In his study of a group of residents from a block of flats in a working-class area of South London, Firth (1956) found that individuals had more extensive knowledge of their kin than first thought. Although people knew little about distant ancestors and could only trace their lineage back to grandparents, they had a remarkably broad knowledge of living relatives. Many of these kin were important in their lives because they were the people they could call on for help in times of crisis. Several of these classic studies demonstrated that membership of extended families was more complex than initially thought. Rather than being static, these kin relationships were adaptable and permeable. Public anxieties about the decline of kinship cohesion were found to be largely misleading.

Nevertheless, the degree of social participation in the past can be overstated because social divisions between people are often overlooked (Devine 1992). Research from the 1950s indicates important gender differences, with women's lives often more home-centred and men's leisure activities typically more communal and located in public areas such as pubs and clubs. This is shown by classic research such as a study of a Yorkshire mining community, *Coal is Our Life*, by Dennis and colleagues (1956). For women, the sense of social isolation was often apparent, given that organized female sociability in public settings was traditionally regulated and restricted. During this period, gender was a major factor affecting people's opportunities for sociable interaction, as well as social class. In terms of class, many forms of working-class employment continue to restrict the time and economic resources needed to engage in various kinds of leisure. However, from the mid twentieth century, the home has become a progressively more socialized space among both working-class and middle-class families (Franklin 1989), especially given the rise in the so-called 'network society' triggered by information technology (Wellman 1979; Chambers 2006). As Allan (1996) states, this trend needs to be taken into account in discussions about the privatization thesis.

Constructions of race in family studies

Research on American families in the 1950s and 1960s was heavily influenced by functionalist theory. As mentioned above, studies tended to elevate the white, middle-class nuclear family as a standard by which all family types were measured (Roschelle 1997). For instance, Parsons (1971) identified African American families as less stable than white nuclear families. Although these families had been disadvantaged by a rigid system of racial stratification, Parsons claimed that they generated 'family disorganization': a weakening of family ties resulting from marital separation and divorce. However, he was criticized for ignoring the resilience and stability of extended kinship networks among Black families, despite the high percentage of female-headed households.

The 'cultural approach' in American family sociology asserted that African Americans and Chicanos attach no special importance to the nuclear family. Instead, they favour the extended kinship network. However, no social or historical explanation was given to clarify why one minority ethnic group might value extended families more than another. This postulation ignored the possibility that an African cultural heritage might characterize the African American family. Extended kinship ties might be an effective way of responding to racism or poverty or might have historical roots in past cultures and places. The unique socio-political histories, migration patterns and cultural norms of the ethnic groups are ignored in this approach (Roschelle 1997). Since the framework of the African American 'culture of poverty' perspective of the 1960s was predicated on the assumption of a white, middle-class, normative model, it underestimated the strength of extended kinship ties. African American family traits such as extended kinship networks were viewed as deviant and disorganized.

The portrayal of African American women as 'matriarchs' encouraged the dominant white group to blame African American women for the poor educational achievements of their children and to ignore racism as a social disadvantage. The social and economic inequalities that disadvantaged African American mothers and their children were sidestepped by the idea that intergenerational poverty was inherited through a pathological family value system. For instance, American sociologist Patrick Moynihan (1965) argued that African American occupational and economic inequality was caused by family disorganization. 'Cultural pathology' was held responsible for the prevalence of female-headed urban families, who were often accused of being 'welfare queens', even though this pattern corresponded with the scarcity of well-paid, secure employment for African American men. A 'culture of poverty' approach towards

Latino families reflected similar ethnocentric, racial prejudice. The privileging of white, middle-class culture encouraged a condemnation of other family forms (Staples and Mirande 1980).

These negative social attributes attached to ethnic minority families in the USA triggered accusations of racism against the 'culture of poverty' approach and the ill-famed report by Moynihan (1965). More liberal academics were reluctant to study minority ethnic families for fear of being labelled racist (Roschelle 1997:6). The rise of poverty, unemployment and social disturbances in urban ghettos of America was overlooked by social scientists for several years after the controversy had subsided (Wilson 1991). Opposing the 'culture of poverty' approach, the 'strength resiliency' perspective emerged in the 1970s to highlight the positive features of African American family life within extended families. This resilience was characterized by the stability of ties between parent and children, informal support networks and the shared community responsibility for children (Aschbrenner 1978). The 'strength resiliency' standpoint embraced cultural relativism by acknowledging the diversity of African American families (Billingsley 1968; Nobles 1974). Nevertheless, this approach continues to overlook the effects of poverty on family organization. The 'adaptive' approach that also countered the 'culture of poverty' approach is also flawed since it tends to idealize the Black mother as powerful, self-reliant and responsible for the endurance of the African American community (McCray 1980).

Similar problems in the sociological study of minority ethnic families occurred in Britain. Caribbean families who migrated to the UK after World War II from the late 1940s deviated from the white middle-class family structure. They were labelled as deviant since it was found that, rather than having patriarchal families headed by a male breadwinner, women played a central role in matrifocal families that lacked male permanent presence (Chamberlain 1999). A high proportion of households headed by single mothers among British African-Caribbean families was correlated with high levels of 'welfare dependency' and social deviance in the community (Dench 1996). Once again, the colonial legacy of slavery and twentieth-century migration were factors neglected in sociological research on minority ethnic families in the UK. From the 1980s and 1990s, the dynamics of migration and the damaging effects of institutional racism and poverty were being uncovered in research on British minority ethnic families (Chamberlain 1995, 1999).

Feminism and families

During the 1970s and 1980s, feminist perspectives led debates and research on the family. The notion of the 'male breadwinner' and the wider patriarchal structure of family life were centrally questioned. The idea that the family is a cooperative unit founded on common interests and mutual support between husband and wife was challenged. The term 'family' itself was perceived as problematic by feminist theories. Monolithic conceptions of the family as a static and unified social grouping were viewed as barriers to understanding the underlying causes of women's oppression in gender relationships (Eichler 1981). Many studies revealed that, despite the idea of the companionate marriage, marriage continued to be an unequal 'partnership' within a highly gendered domestic division of labour (Oakley 1974; Delphy 1977; Edgell 1980; Mansfield and Collard 1987; Delphy and Leonard 1992). The occurrence of domestic violence and high levels of divorce highlighted the discrepancy between the ideals and realities of marriage. By the 1990s, almost half of marriages were ending in separation in the USA, UK and other western nations (Allan 1996).

Barrett and McIntosh (1982) identified the term 'family' as a form of ideology rather than simply a descriptive concept. They regarded 'the family' as a set of values that maintains women's subordination. Dissatisfaction among wives was undermined by appealing to the 'naturalness' of the biological unit of the heterosexual couple and their children. The work of Barrett and McIntosh initiated new approaches in which the term 'family' was replaced by more useful terms such as 'households', to encourage the ideology of the family to be interrogated rather than naturalized. By shifting the focus of attention, feminists were able to address the inequalities experienced by women in marriage and their family lives. Whether or not the family reinforces patriarchy or capitalism or some other system beyond the family was examined, following the work of Engels (see, for example, Coward 1983). From the 1970s, feminist scholars argued that gender inequalities were being deflected by claims that the patriarchal structure of the heterosexual family was innate. New ways of analysing the family were combined with Marxist ideas. Feminist perspectives provided interconnected critiques of the linked social conditions that caused inequalities of gender in the home, in the labour market and in poverty after divorce (Firestone 1970; Greer 1970; Millet 1970; Mitchell 1975; Barrett 1980).

Feminist sociologists advanced debates about the socially constructed nature of family life by focusing on the way domestic tasks such as childcare and housework are divided between men and women. A range of work challenged the validity of assertions of the 'symmetrical family' by Young and Willmott (1957, 1987) in their study of kinship in East London. This concept described the idea that husbands and wives were more equal since they shared domestic roles and responsibilities more fairly. Arguing for more rigorous research on gender relationships, Ann Oakley (1974) legitimized the academic study of domestic work at a time when housework had not been considered worthy of study in sociology because it was such a routine and private activity. The domestic sphere of labour had been marginalized and rendered invisible. Even though women are now engaged in paid employment outside the home in larger numbers than ever before, research confirms that wives still endure the main responsibility for domestic work and have less leisure time at their disposal than their husbands, as the following chapters show (Hochschild 1989; Gershuny et al. 1994; Sullivan 2000).

Feminist research highlighted the ways in which childhood socialization into traditional sex roles corresponds with different social experiences for men and women from cradle to grave. For example, the apparently more physical and energetic behaviour of boys and more caring and obedient behaviour of girls were exposed as gender stereotypes that regulate children's behaviour. Studies were conducted on the ways in which these distinctions are rationalized into sexist ideologies that claim gender differences are natural (Oakley 1972; Stanley and Wise 1983). For example, the maternal deprivation thesis advanced by professionals such as John Bowlby (1953) elevated the mystique of the emotional and psychological bonding between mother and child, promoting the idea that working women do not make good mothers. A separation from the mother, when the child is cared for by another relative such as the grandmother, was seen to have an adverse effect on the child. This view furthered women's confinement to the home and ignored the significance of other kin and community support in childcare. It also deterred the state from providing childcare for working mothers. Theories of maternal deprivation which underlined women's primary role as carers in the functional nuclear family were critiqued by feminist perspectives as ideologies of 'bad mothering' (Davidoff et al. 1999).

Feminist scholarship also drew attention to the gender segregation of the labour market as a way in which gendered roles in the family are naturalized in paid labour. The treatment of women as a 'reserve army of labour' to be used in times of labour shortages or war, and of their wages as 'pin money', for superfluous luxuries, was propelled by the idea of women's employment as a sideline to husbands' wages. Feminists pointed out that the family is founded on gendered differences reflected and perpetuated in a labour market. Women tend to be channelled into low-paid 'feminized labour' that reflects the domestic and childcare tasks assigned to women, such as nursing, teaching and catering (see Oakley 1974; Hartmann 1976; Gamarnikow 1985; Walby 1985; Delphy and Leonard 1992; Woodroffe 2009). Women are often discriminated against in highly paid professional and managerial careers where they confront a 'glass ceiling' due to their assumed childrearing role (see Rake and Lewis 2009). The unequal distribution of resources among family members and the control of and access to family finances by husbands have also been publicized through feminist research (Pahl 1989).

Feminist scholarship of the 1970s and 1980s also examined the way the family serves as a context for gender oppression and physical abuse. Violence in the home, including 'wife battering', marital rape and child abuse, was once routinely ignored but was now being uncovered through feminist research. The prevalent idea that the home is a safe haven for children, women and older people was challenged (Dobash and Dobash 1980, 1992). Domestic violence, child abuse, divorce, widowhood, mental and physical health problems, poverty and homelessness were exposed (see Dallos and McLaughlin, 1993). Feminist writing on the family in the 1970s and 1980s was, then, diverse in terms of political and theoretical objectives and extensive in its empirical emphases. Its contributions to the sociology of the family were so fundamental that it comprised a set of overriding critiques of conventional sociological views of family life as harmonious and egalitarian (Smart 2007). The family was no longer viewed as sacrosanct or inevitably functional for its members. Feminists pointed out that men benefited from family life more than women.

Feminist work also contributed to the foundations of queer theory by questioning the naturalness of the heterosexual relationships on which family life is founded and by exposing the historical and cultural labelling of alternatives to heterosexuality as deviant (for example, Rich 1980; Weeks 1985). In the 1950s and 1960s, all other forms of intimacy that did not conform to heterosexual marriage and family life were perceived as inferior or deviant (Rosenfeld 1999; Holden 2007; Porche and Purvin 2008). In Britain, male homosexuality was illegal until 1967. In the USA , homosexuality was defined as a mental disorder until as late as 1973 by the American Psychological Association. Under these circumstances, men and women felt pressured to conceal their sexual identities, with some feeling pressured to marry (Rosenfeld 1999). Legal recognition of non-heterosexual relationships took place in 2005 in Britain, when civil registrations were introduced. The history is more complicated in the USA since it differs from state to state, with Massachusetts being the first to authorize same-sex marriage in 2004. Feminist and gay and lesbian scholarship questioned the dominant *heteronormative* and *patriarchal* social order challenged by gay and lesbian relationships (Dalton and Bielby 2000). 'Heteronormative' is a term used in queer theory, introduced by Michael Warner (1991), to describe the expectations, social pressures and constraints exerted on individuals when heterosexuality is taken as the norm in society. The influence of gay and lesbian studies on the sociology of the family is addressed in the following chapter.

Conclusions

This chapter has shown how the roots of some of today's enduring ideas about the family lie within the work of classical thinkers. It demonstrates how late nineteenth-century and early twentieth-century sociological theories about the family contributed to or sustained biological and social discourses, often drawing on quite contradictory frameworks of thinking. On the one hand, the family was assumed to be a universal *biological* unit. On the other hand, sociologists were preoccupied with the effects of *social* and *economic* change on family structures. Although the family was mainly viewed through a biological lens, it was a lens used selectively to authenticate and legitimate an approved, monogamous, patriarchal, nuclear version sanctioned by a companionate partnership. A second area of concern for sociologists was with the effects of industrialization and urbanization on family structures and the desire to elevate a recent, nuclear model as the norm. A major and continuing issue for both academics and governments was the fear that the family unit was in a state of decline, being compromised by encroaching individualism and privatization. The ideal companionate marriage was promoted to strengthen modern conjugal relationships in the light of a decline in traditional community. Based on positive intimate relationships between partners, it acted as proof that the 'modern marriage' was becoming more egalitarian. By narrowly defining a small, mobile nuclear family as universal, functionalism treated all other family types as deviations.

The fact that the nuclear family was neither universal nor permanent was repeatedly confirmed by statistical evidence in western societies. Dramatic changes in family structures were taking place across the twentieth century. Parsons did not predict the rise of divorce and separation among white, middle-class families by the end of the twentieth century. In the United States, the number of households with two parents and children declined by 20 per cent between the 1960s and 1990s (Casper and Bianchi 2002:11 and 99). Since the 1950s, the number of children in single-parent households in the USA has risen significantly. In 1950, 93 per cent of children lived in a nuclear family, while only 6 per cent lived with their mother and 1 per cent with their father. By 1998, 73 per cent lived in a nuclear family, 22 per cent with their mother and 5 per cent with their father. Moreover, many families that appeared to be nuclear were reconstituted families after divorce and remarriage. White couples in the USA are increasingly likely to live in households without children (Casper and Bianchi 2002:99). While the majority of Americans were married by the age of twenty-five in 1960, by 1998 around half of all men and 40 per cent of women remained unmarried by this age. This change coincided with a rise in cohabitation. In 1978 only 3 per cent of women and 4 per cent of men cohabited. By 1998, 9 per cent of women and 12 per cent of men did so (Casper and Bianchi 2002:42).

These figures indicate that attitudes and behaviour changed dramatically in a short time from the middle to the end of the twentieth century. Yet certain values and practices persist. The next chapter addresses recent research which demonstrates the importance of continuity and connectedness among family members. One of the major distinctions between traditional and more recent approaches to the family is the shift away from the idea of 'the family' as a *social institution* governed by rigid moral conventions to an idea of family and wider personal life as diverse sets of *practices*. The following chapters indicate that the focus today, in sociological debates, is on interactive processes and the agency of individuals and family members in relation to the social constraints of gender, social class, race and migration.

2 Individualization, Intimacy and Family Life

Having considered late nineteenth- to mid-twentieth-century debates about family life, this chapter focuses on new social theories from the 1990s that have become highly influential. Claims are made that we have entered a new, more democratic phase of family life from the late twentieth century. New versions of 'family' are said to have been generated by key changes in ideas about love and commitment. However, many of the concerns about family decline expressed in the nineteenth and twentieth centuries are still present in late modern social theory. The increasing diversity of contemporary family forms – including same-sex couples, single-parent families, and post-divorce families – has prompted anxieties about the wider social trends and underlying social conditions that correspond with new kinds of personal relationships. These transformations in family life are said to be part of an erosion of traditional forms of the collective solidarity that once characterized extended kinship and community networks. The *individualization thesis* aims to explain the changes, exemplified by the work of Giddens (1992), Beck and Beck-Gernsheim (1995) and Bauman (2003).

The new ideas about love and intimate life are traced in this chapter in relation to the changing nature of the self and society. Alternative approaches to family studies are considered by looking at the contributions made by concepts such as 'family practices' and 'displaying families' to debates about the family. Critiques of late modern social theory are then addressed by assessing recent empirical evidence about alternative and diverse family forms, including same-sex couples and the use of terms such as 'families of choice' to express the formation and meanings of lesbian and gay families. Patterns of family life among minority ethnic families, including intergenerational ties, are then focused on.

Individualization and changing families

The concept of individualization has been used by social theorists from the 1990s to explain major changes in the family from the mid twentieth century onwards. The individualization thesis, also referred to as 'de-traditionalization', explains a revision of the boundaries between femininity and masculinity, including changes in the roles of motherhood, fatherhood and childhood. Up to the mid twentieth century, family life was more strongly regulated, with roles prescribed by gender. The assumption was that husbands worked outside the home and wives took responsibility for childcare and domestic work. Women were expected to give up employment when they married. The individualization thesis draws attention to the weakening of these traditional customs which once bound families together. It foregrounds a corresponding rise in individual agency and personal choice. We are entering a new stage of family life which Giddens describes as the 'democratic' family (Giddens 1992).

Individualization involves the erosion of traditional values and the rise of individual agency (Giddens 1992, 1998; Beck 1992, 1994). Contemporary changes in family life are coinciding with social and geographical mobility, and shifts in employment and in class identities. New kinds of lifestyles emphasize the agency and autonomy of the individual. Based on consumerism, new lifestyles seem to offer a wider range of choices about how to live one's life. One of the general outcomes of these changes is that social categories such as 'gender' and 'sexuality', which were once regarded as biologically determined, are being contested and transformed. At the same time, intimacy is being transformed from a set of social obligations and conventions to a new kind of *democracy* between couples. Inequality may continue to exist in personal relationships, but late modern theory suggests that this is more effectively explained at the level of the individual rather than in terms of a particular group or class. How family members understand their social position and their interactions with other people is guided less by traditional duties and more by active choice and negotiation between individuals.

For Giddens (1992), a feature of contemporary marital relationships that distinguishes them from those of previous decades is the idea of *confluent love* and the *pure relationship*. 'Confluent love' is an active and contingent love, in which intimate relationships are characterized by personal understandings between two people. This kind of association is identified as a 'pure relationship' since the relationship is developed by the couple for its own sake. It is shaped by an attachment of trust and emotional interaction rather than by external pressures such as the demands of parents and wider kin, as in arranged marriages, or by other external standards and values. Giddens defined a pure relationship as conditional, in the sense of it being conditional on both parties wanting the relationship to continue. It is a relationship which is maintained until further notice, on condition that it is reciprocally fulfilling. He states:

> A pure relationship has nothing to do with sexual purity, and is a limiting concept rather than only a descriptive one. It refers to a situation where a social relation is entered into for its own sake, for what can be derived by each person from a sustained association with another; and which is continued only in so far as it is thought by both parties to deliver enough satisfactions for each individual to stay within it. (Giddens 1992:58)

The confluent love involved in this pure relationship is described as dynamic, conditional love. It is not necessarily 'forever' in the same way as traditional ideas of marital love:

> Confluent love is active, contingent love, and therefore jars with the 'for-ever', 'one-and-only' qualities of the romantic love complex. The 'separating and divorcing society' of today here appears as an effect of the emergence of confluent love rather than its cause. (Giddens 1992:61)

To some extent, this progress made in heterosexual relationships can be viewed as a revision of the 'companionate marriage', discussed in chapter 1. However, according to Giddens (1992:61), these changes have been propelled by 'the pressure of female sexual emancipation and autonomy' and are accompanied by problems. The emphasis on romantic love linked with a project of the self coincides with a crisis of moral commitment. These changes in love have exposed the provisional nature of commitment between couples. They also give rise to new challenges in providing stable and sustained childcare. Individualism seems, then, to conflict with the needs of the family, with the former emphasizing individual choice and the latter relying on commitment, stability and permanence. The new emphasis on individual choice and self-fulfilment has created new *risks* as well as *opportunities* (Beck 1992; Beck and Beck-Gernsheim 1995, 2002). New opportunities are generated by less rigid gender roles and the rise of more flexible and egalitarian relationships between couples. This flexibility involves a tolerance for alternative and more experimental intimacies such as cohabitation, living apart but together (LATS), and lesbian and gay relationships.

These new life experiments are risky since they are often characterized by temporary and transient relationships, as indicated by rising divorce rates. Intimate relationships are no longer controlled by rigid rules. Instead, they involve negotiation and bargaining. The old certainties of eternal love have withered away yet continue to be yearned for. And the old assurances of 'knowing your place' in the world are replaced by a new self-reflexivity in which individuals must now actively work at constructing their identities through the project of the 'self'. With former rules and structures no longer shaping their lives, individuals must invent their own biographies and life projects. Personal agency is said to be gaining a new significance through the personal negotiation and management of one's life events (Giddens 1991, 1992; Beck and Beck-Gernsheim 2002). Today's reflexive project of the self is linked to the sphere of intimacy in which romantic love shapes the narrative in individuals' lives. This change is viewed negatively. It makes the project of the self all the more challenging and precarious, given that romance may be temporary.

The degree of personal choice and agency in late modernity provokes problems in sexual relationships. Practical self-help guides now offer us advice, counselling and lifestyle philosophies to help us create or re-invent our life narratives, to tackle the crises and insecurities thrown up by today's apparently more volatile and unpredictable life trajectories. A string of book titles provides clues of the kinds of themes that we are expected to be preoccupied with, such as *Relate Guide to Staying Together. From Crisis to Deeper Commitment* (Quilliam 1995) and *Loving Yourself Loving Another: The Importance of Self-esteem for Successful Relationships* (Cole 2001). One of the bestsellers, *Men Are from Mars, Women Are from Venus* (Gray 2002) is tellingly subtitled: *A Practical Guide for Improving Communication and Getting What You Want in Your Relationships*. We are expected to be preoccupied with our *selves* and our *personal* relationships within a rising tide of narcissism (Lasch 1979).

The challenges of handling intimate relationships in these times of apparent uncertainty are topics that also saturate lifestyle magazines and webzines and they even masquerade in newspapers as 'news', especially when associated with the love lives of celebrities. A whole industry has developed around the self-help discourse, leading to the rise of therapy news and self-confessional journalism (Chambers et al. 2004a). In addition to practical self-help guides on how to create a stable self-narrative and handle our personal and family relationships, we are offered advice on broader life philosophies to help us steer our way through the confusing range of lifestyle choices. Once guided by the values of the religion of our parents, we are now able to consider alternatives: vegetarianism, Buddhism, New Age spiritualism, and mental and spiritual healing as examples of a bewildering array of lifestyle options and philosophies in narrating our individual identities.

Notwithstanding the risks entailed in the contingent nature of today's relationships in terms of commitment, Giddens argues that intimate ties between men and women are also being transformed in *positive* ways. He emphasizes the importance of same-sex relationships which he claims are at the vanguard of these new, democratic relationships. Gay and lesbian intimacies tend to question and break away from traditional roles of obligation. They create the possibility of reclassifying and modernizing relationships as egalitarian. He refers to same-sex relationships as 'prime everyday experimenters'. However, Giddens has been criticized for overlooking differential relations of power in terms of social class, gender inequality and intergenerational connections (Jamieson 1999; Smart and Neale 1999; Crow 2002; Ribbens McCarthy and Edwards 2002; Smart 2007). Indeed, there is sparse evidence to support the claim that the democratic 'pure relationship' has been achieved, as Lynn Jamieson (1999) points out. Nevertheless, the use of the notion of the democratic relationship in today's intimate ties is symptomatic of important *aspirations* towards equality and mutual understanding, especially by women who seek more balanced and equal partnerships with their partners. Thus, in defence, Giddens argues that he is identifying an ideal type or emergent family association which is anticipated and which may evolve in the future.

Elizabeth Beck-Gernsheim (2002) argues that although individuals now have more personal choice in deciding how to shape their lives, relationships have become thinner, more fragile and more temporary. For Ulrich Beck (1992), this is a contradiction of the late modern condition. On the one hand, men and women are freed from traditional constraints and ascribed roles, and are now authors of their own lives. On the other hand, the weakening of social ties compels people to bond in the pursuit of romantic fulfilment in order to avoid loneliness. The yearning for a mutual intimate life is signified by the idyll of romantic attachment and marital union. The work on individualization by Beck and Beck-Gernsheim (1995, 2002) is, then, more pessimistic than that of Giddens. They argue that families are gradually fragmenting as a result of social conditions associated with the atomization of self-absorbed individuals.

The kinds of conditions that correspond with this fragmentation and atomization include women's employment, gender equality and the demand for more flexibility and mobility both in labour markets and in intimate lives. Yet, rather than prompting individuals to turn their backs on marriage and procreation, these dramatic social changes encourage individuals to search for constancy and security through intimacy. Finding romance becomes progressively more urgent as the failures of individualization mount in the wake of its rising hopes and possibilities (Beck 1992:105). Love is viewed as the only condition that can give meaning to our lives. Yet, paradoxically, the lack of firm foundations to family life means that individuals are finding it increasingly difficult to sustain these kinds of intimate relationships. This leads to escalating divorce rates. Beck and Beck-Gernsheim (1995:173) assert that, at the very moment that the family is spiralling into disintegration, it is being placed on a pedestal, treated as sacred. As a result, both sexes set their standards too high and are inevitably disappointed. During a time when long-term commitment between adults is eroding, children are focused on as providers of a more permanent love.

Zygmunt Bauman's work on the family echoes the pessimism of Beck and Beck-Gernsheim's approach. In his book *Liquid Love* (2003), Bauman interprets the decline in fixed kinship systems and ascribed roles and ascent of elective kinship affinity as a negative change. He emphasizes the frailty of contemporary family bonds and argues that the ill-defined nature of family roles is jeopardizing the family as an institution. Growing disagreements about property title and inheritance between couples are highlighted by Bauman as examples of problems in this respect. However, he offers no concrete empirical evidence to support his argument.

These late modern theories of changing family life have been criticized on several levels. A number of academics have drawn attention to discrepancies between the kind of 'family' portrayed by the individualization thesis and the complex family lives documented in today's small-scale empirical studies about family, kinship and friendship from the late twentieth century onwards (Jamieson 1998; Lewis,

2001; Crow 2002; Ribbens McCarthy et al. 2003; Smart and Shipman 2004; Brannen and Nilsen 2005; Gross 2005; Duncan and Smith 2006; Smart 2007). First, these grand theories about family life in late modernity appear somewhat abstracted from everyday lives in real contexts. Second, and related to this problem of abstraction, Giddens (1990) and Beck and Beck-Gernsheim (2002) have been criticized for exaggerating individual choice. They give too much weight to the idea of individuals as active agents, thereby viewing people's actions as the outcome of personal choice (Williams 2008:491). For example, Giddens tends to perceive heterosexual couples as free to negotiate the conditions of their relationship as if they were unconstrained by today's gendered relations and class structures. This is indicated by his concept of the 'pure relationship' (Jamieson 1999). This tendency also characterizes the work of Beck and Beck-Gernsheim. Bauman (2003) presents even more fluid individual choices compared to the combination of structure and agency in the reflexive thesis of Giddens and Beck and Beck-Gernsheim (Williams 2008:492). Third, one of the consequences of this over-determination of individual agency is that these late modern theorists suffer from a lack of awareness of gender and social class constraints in family life. Fourth, the fears and constraints associated with homophobia for lesbian and gay couples also tend to be underplayed.

Notwithstanding these drawbacks, Giddens' approach to the changing nature and meaning of 'family' life in the last couple of decades is less negative than that of Bauman (2003) and Beck and Beck-Gernsheim (1995). He embraces features of familial change, emphasizing the importance of same-sex relationships. The discretionary and flexible nature of family relationships tends to be resented by Bauman and by Beck and Beck-Gernsheim. Giddens praises the emergence of the democratic relationship while Beck and Beck-Gernsheim criticize this new kind of relationship for being unachievable and for giving rise to the disappointments and tensions in marriage. The latter assert the impossibility of the family as an egalitarian institution (Smart 2007:19).

A major problem for the sociology of the family is that, although the individualization thesis is criticized for not being informed by empirical research data, these ideas are popular in the public sphere and are shaping political debates about family life. Politicians and the media are drawing on and exaggerating accounts of a 'decline' of 'proper' family life. Late modern theories of the family are perceived by some critics to be reflecting populist thinking (Smart 2004, 2007; see chapter 9). While the stress on individual agency and choice assumes equality between men and women, a normative assumption persists that caring roles should still mainly be the responsibility of women, rather than a joint responsibility between men and women. This view also presupposes that family life in general is being undermined by women, children are being uncared for and older family members left vulnerable in old age. The resentment is driven, then, by women's personal autonomy and their apparently successful movement into employment. Women are thought to have too much choice. They are regarded as self-interested agents.

Doing and displaying families

A key challenge for the sociology of the family has, then, been the need for empirical research and concepts sufficiently sensitive to identify and explain the complexities and diversity of family life. From the 1990s, new ways of thinking beyond or in response to the 'individualization' thesis have advanced studies of families, relationships and kinship. A key example is David Morgan's concept of 'family practices' (Morgan 1996, 2011). Morgan's 'practices' approach is based on the recognition of a mismatch between the ideological notion of the nuclear family and the variety of ways in which real people conduct their family lives. The idea of understanding how people actually 'do family life' provides a useful way to explore the complex realities of family living. His work has extended the field conceptually by highlighting the need to define families by their *customs* and *practices* rather than exclusively by co-residence or even simply by kinship and marriage.

Morgan explains that family members are 'social actors' who engage in the actions and activities that comprise the routines of doing family life. The emphasis is on how people 'do' relationships, parenthood and kinship. He points out that, by emphasizing the performance of family life, we can go beyond the unproductive discussion about whether the institution of 'the family' is declining or not. By drawing attention to family *practices* rather than family *structures*, a wide range of personal relationships can be recognized and accepted as having equal legitimacy. Whether the partnership is a same-sex or a heterosexual union or whether it entails marriage or cohabitation is not the main issue. This approach therefore allows us to understand diverse and experimental family forms, such as gay and lesbian families. For example, Christopher Carrington (1999) uses the term 'doing family life' to explain the ways in which many gay and lesbian couples' relationships are negotiated. Morgan also uses the concept of 'family practices' for an understanding of heterosexual couples by emphasizing the *performativity* of family life in general. Morgan acknowledges the inclusion of more diverse, multi-faceted and fluid relationships that are family-like, including friendships (see chapter 9). The 'doing' of family life becomes more significant than the institutional and legal framework in which it is set.

For Morgan, alternatives to 'family', and a broadening of the term, include 'intimacy', 'personal life', the 'total social organization of labour' and 'caringscapes'. These terms are chosen to prevent a nuclear version of 'family' from being exclusionary. However, Morgan (2011) argues that the term 'family' should not be abandoned. It remains meaningful and the term 'family practices' is sufficiently fluid to embrace intimate and personal practices. Although the concept of 'intimacy' is linked with Giddens' work on transformation of intimacy in late modernity, Morgan, instead, draws on the approach of Lynn Jamieson (1998). He argues that, while Giddens' perspective is fairly optimistic, Jamieson offers an analysis based on historical and empirical evidence. She uses the term 'disclosing intimacy' to describe an intimacy of the self rather than a sexual intimacy. This allows the term to be used to explain changes in parent–child relationships. Today's parent–child relationships are characterized by 'disclosing intimacy'. Morgan also highlights the importance of emotions to family practices. Academic research is not only increasingly foregrounding the emotional work involved in sexual intimacies and for women in duties of care. It is also highlighting the structuring of wider caring economies through emotional exchanges in women's paid employment as nurses, carers, nannies and domestic cleaners (for example, Nelson 1998; Hochschild 2003b; Zelizer 2005; see chapters 6 and 9). Morgan's work on family practices represents, then, a shift of focus from the family as an *institution* to a set of *social practices*.

The concept of family practices has been used in various studies, including research by Smart and Neale (1999), to explain the family dynamics that follow divorce. Former partners find themselves engaged in the shared parenting of their children in a new kind of 'divorced parenting' partnership which calls for them to be 'separate yet connected' (1999:67). This kind of post-divorce co-parenting disrupts the conventions of nuclear families. Divorced parents find themselves in 'chains of relationships' with several individuals and across households (1999:72). By using the concept of 'family practices', Smart and Neale have considered how people *practise* family life under circumstances brought about by divorce which, at various points in time, involve different partners and different groupings of children. For people involved in co-parenting, the need to demonstrate that one is engaged in 'good parenting' is paramount (see chapter 3). The probability that a person will be a 'good parent' can influence legal conclusions during a divorce. Smart and Neale found that exhibiting 'good parenting' also has ongoing legal and moral importance. Thus, the public *performance* of good parenting practice has profound consequences in a legal context. It determines whether a parent will have or be denied contact with their child.

Further research work, carried out by the CAVA research programme on 'Care, Values and the Future of Welfare'[1] at Leeds University between 1999 and 2004, demonstrates that the group of people that we identify as 'my family' is no longer necessarily the same as those living in our own household. Many people experience close relationships that stretch out beyond their own to other households as a result of divorce, step-parents and children, cohabitation, and wider family relationships, and through same-sex partnerships and friendships. These links may even traverse countries and continents via migration processes (Williams 2004; see chapter 6).

Janet Finch (2007) has extended Morgan's 'family practices' approach by suggesting that families should not simply be equated with households. Families need to be *displayed* as well as practised. Finch (2007:67) states that 'Display is the process by which individuals, and groups of individuals, convey to each other and to relevant audiences that certain of their actions do constitute "doing family things" and thereby confirm that these relationships are "family" relationships.' Finch emphasizes the importance of social interactions, particularly the ways in which social meanings about the 'family-like' nature of one's relationships are conveyed to, understood and supported by relevant others. Rituals such as family meals, family photographs, weddings and funerals are compelling modes of display which convey powerful meanings of family togetherness.

Finch (2007) identifies narratives, stories about family and personal or domestic objects as major tools for displaying family and kin relationships. People create stories to explain to themselves and to others their family and kin relationships. Finch (2007:79) emphasizes that individuals are compelled to display and narrate relationships to publicly confirm their existence or success. She outlines situations in which the need for display becomes more intense as a result of changed family circumstances. An example of an indirect form of display is the presentation of photographs in people's homes, which can convey and reinforce meanings about relationships. While display work is clearly relevant in general to families and intimacies, Finch also suggests that display may be more significant for those people who live in families which do *not* fit conventional ideas of what a 'proper' family looks like. For instance, the concept of display has proved to be important for an understanding of gay and lesbian families where the trappings of normal family life, such as putting family photos on show in the home, form key roles in demonstrating the commitment between the couple (see Weeks et al. 2001).

Finch's (2007) notion of 'displaying families' is used by Kathryn Almack (2008) to examine how narratives about 'coming out' are used when lesbian couples become parents. Almack explains how 'family display' was drawn on as a resource by the lesbian couples in her study:

> It highlights how, for many respondents in my study, having a child required the need to actively negotiate and demonstrate familial relationships with their families of origin. This includes the working out of new kin relationships between their child and their families of origin, the extent to which these relationships were recognized and validated, and also a consideration of the extent to which family members come out about the lesbian parent family within their own networks. (Almack 2008:1194–5)

This display work confirmed the depth of the couples' commitment to sustaining family and wider kin relationships. Photographs were mentioned as a meaningful sign of the level of acceptance of their new family by their family of origin and of the degree to which their family of origin felt at ease about admitting the lesbian parent family to others within their own networks. Late modern theories and public assessments of contemporary intimate relationships tend to perceive families as unstable, with individuals putting their own interests first, leading to a loss of commitment to family relationships. Yet these findings contradict such perspectives. Instead, Almack found that many of her respondents worked hard to maintain close relationships with their families of origin even when they had been let down and disappointed by an absence of familial display work by their relatives. Their accounts demonstrated a deep commitment to their families of origin (see also Dunne 2000). This concurs with the conclusions arrived at by Fiona Williams (2004) in her summary of the collection of research by CAVA. Almack's findings contribute to a growing body of evidence that indicates that people are 'energetic moral actors, embedded in webs of valued personal relationships, working to sustain the commitments that matter to them' (Williams 2004:41, quoted in Almack 2008:1195). Importantly, then, this kind of small-scale research on the display work of same-sex couples suggests that fears of a decline of commitment in the individualization thesis are unfounded.

'Unconventional' family relationships

As we have seen, the growing trend of heterosexual couples living together without or before marrying is viewed negatively by some commentators on 'the family'. Cohabitation is often viewed as evidence of a decline in the willingness to invest in permanent partnerships. However, other sociological studies have questioned the link between increasing cohabitation and a declining commitment to life-long partnerships. Assumptions that cohabitation involves less commitment than more traditional long-term relationships have not been confirmed through empirical research (Prinz 1995; Manting 1996; Lewis 1999, 2001; Lewis et al. 1999; Ermisch 2000; Smart and Stevens 2000). Instead, recent empirical work has arrived at a more nuanced interpretation of family and personal relationships. Conclusions differ about the extent to which individuals are engaged in 'everyday social experiments' (Jamieson 1998; Lewis 1999; Smart and Neale 1999; Ribbens McCarthy et al. 2003). Indeed, the use of the term 'commitment' to describe intimate relationships is very recent. It originates from the late twentieth century. A study by Jane Lewis (Lewis et al.1999) shows that the term 'obligation' was more widely used by the older generation and the word 'commitment' by the younger generation (1999b:44).

Lewis proposes that, for more recent generations, the *moral* distinction between marriage and cohabitation no longer exists. Younger people nowadays tend to believe that the commitment made by couples to each other is 'their own affair' (2001:145). Other academics predict that attitudes to cohabitation will gradually shift from being viewed as a *preface* to marriage to being viewed as an acceptable *alternative* union (Haskey 1999, 2001; Kiernan 1999). These views seem to be supported by research evidence. A study of partnership formation in the Netherlands since the 1950s by Dorien Manting (1996) indicates that cohabitation begins as an alternative way of living, then shifts to an interim phase before marriage, and ultimately becomes a plan for moving gradually into a permanent union.

Further research on cohabiting by Lynn Jamieson et al. (2002) found no simple correspondence between cohabiting and 'lack of commitment'. Over 200 heterosexual couples aged twenty to twenty-nine were included in their British study – a key age group in terms of ideals and practices of partnership formation. A strong commitment by couples to long-term or life-time partnering was revealed. This refutes the pessimistic view that a rise in cohabitation demonstrates a selfish unwillingness to commit to long-term family relationships. Survey data and in-depth interviews indicated that most couples described living together as the start of a permanent arrangement. Couples supported cohabitation because they believed that marriage would 'make no difference' or because they 'had not yet got round to' marriage. However, the idea that 'marriage is better for children' continued to be upheld by respondents. On average, cohabiting couples had lower incomes and poorer employment situations than married couples, but only extreme adverse circumstances were viewed as a barrier or risk to marriage (Jamieson et al. 2002).

A study in the United States of three-generation families by Vern Bengtson et al. (2002) found that feelings of solidarity and closeness with parents have not changed between generations. The findings indicated that young people today have as much affection and regard for their parents as their parents did for theirs. Divorce or mothers' employment does not noticeably affect the well-being of the child. Working mothers invest the same amount of emotional and material resources in their children as previous generations of mothers who were not in paid employment. Researchers concluded that families continue to be of importance to children, providing no evidence that the family is in decline. Nevertheless, the authors stressed that families are not static and should not be idealized. Rather, they see families as changing, adjusting to social conditions around them. Resonating with Morgan's (1996) work on family practices and emphasis on 'doing' relationships rather than on structures and status, Bengtson et al. (2002) emphasize that families are defined by what they *do*.

The manner in which the late modern family is being portrayed by the individualization thesis is further questioned by findings of a small-scale study of parenting and step-parenting in the UK by Ribbens McCarthy, Edwards and Gillies (2003). In forty-six in-depth interviews of twenty-three stepfamilies, family members did not see family, partnership and kinship as conditional or tempo-rary. Yet couples in stepfamilies are precisely the kinds of unions identified by the individualization thesis as being characterized by autonomous, self-reflexive individuals who view relationships as conditional and transient. Instead, these researchers discovered that couples and their children generated what they call a 'community of need' in which they gave priority to support and duty between family members. Rather than uncovering evidence of moral diversity,   · these researchers found that parents gave priority to their children's needs and, in doing so, were guided by strong moral certainties. Class and gender influenced parents' inclination to demonstrate that they put their children first. Working-class families tended to meet their children's needs by reassembling a non-biological family in *one household*. Among middle-class parents, children's needs were addressed by maintaining the biological family *across households*. Thus, the construction of the stepfamily was motivated by a sense of duty in caring for the children. Again, the researchers found no confirmation of couples pursuing relationships of a democratic but ephemeral nature. Instead, most couples sought to be in 'normal' families with committed, enduring relationships. This work concurs with other research on moral values associated with family and kinship obligations (Williams 2004).

Same-sex intimacies and families of choice

In a world of changing relationships, the continuing use of the word 'family' seems to suggest the power and flexibility of this concept. It is being used to include a range of associations and households that would not have fitted Talcott Parson's narrow sociological definition of a nuclear family in the 1950s (chapter 1). The concept of *families of choice* (Weston 1991) and of *friends as family* (Spencer and Pahl 2006) evolved as a result of a now more *inclusive* definition of 'family'. These concepts, of 'friendship' and 'friends as family', are also explored in more detail in the final chapter for an understanding of the increasing diversity and fluidity of intimate relationships in contemporary societies. As we have seen, a growing number of studies focus on the family lives of same-sex couples (for example Dunne 2000; Weeks et al. 2001; Gabb 2004). The idea that individuals are making their own choices rather than feeling compelled to follow rigid customs associated with responsibility and obligation has particular resonance for gay and lesbian couples. Sociological debates about the increasing *diversity* of family lives have been particularly influenced by the individualization thesis. For example, Giddens' work has been of value to those researching same-sex relationships (Weeks et al. 2001). As mentioned, Giddens (1992:135) suggests that those in same-sex relationships are at the vanguard of these changes. Jeffrey Weeks and colleagues (2001) concur that 'non-heterosexuals' are leading wider changes to family lives. This emphasis has given rise to the theorizing of lesbian, gay and bisexual relational configurations as 'families of choice' (Weeks et al. 2001; Weston 1991). But are these new configurations of intimate life transcending the *gendered* organization of domestic routines?

Gillian Dunne (1997) refers to the prescribed *gender scripts* in relationships in the context of 'institutional heterosexuality'. These gender scripts are employed to negotiate or guide interaction. However, Dunne states that in gay, lesbian and bisexual relationships, many of the features of conventional domestic practices are disrupted. One of the most valued aspects of lesbian lifestyles, by those in a lesbian relationship, is the achievement of an egalitarian relationship (Peplau and Cochran 1990; Johnson 1990; Dunne 1997; Weeks et al. 1999b, 2001). However, the dynamics of same-sex relationships can often be complicated by one or both partners' previous experiences of marriage which can generate expectations about the criteria for successful or failed relationships. For example, as in heterosexual relationships, differences in income or status of employment and unequal contribution to domestic work, parenting and caring all have the potential to generate tensions in the relationship.

As Carrington (1999) argues, there is an assumption among some commentators that the traditional assignment of domestic tasks on the basis of gender does not occur among lesbian, gay and bisexual couples. Nevertheless, gay and lesbian couples still have to negotiate the potentially challenging problems of domesticity. Evidence of tension about the allocation of household tasks among gay and lesbian couples in his ethnographic study convinces Carrington that they are no different from heterosexual couples. He states:

> My research seriously challenges the effort to place the lesbigay family in the vanguard of social change, a model of equality for others to emulate. Such assertions are based on the ideology of egalitarianism, not on its actual existence, and on the invisibility, devaluation, and diminishment of domesticity. (1999:218)

Notwithstanding the fact that domestic tasks are undertaken inequitably in some gay and lesbian households, many gay and lesbian couples do believe they have achieved equality in relationships (Carrington 1999).

'Families of choice' may include relationships based on blood ties and can also encompass relationships founded on friendships. These friendship relationships become 'family-like' in terms of levels of commitment and support. Weeks et al. (2001:8) suggest that non-heterosexual parenting is 'probably the most controversial and contested aspect of families of choice'. Findings indicate an increasing public tolerance of same-sex relationships but not the same level of acceptance of same-sex parenting (Duncan and Phillips 2008). 'Families of choice' was a term adopted by friends and by gay and lesbian couples to valorize non-heterosexual relationships (Weeks et al. 2001). Weeks et al. (2001) point out that the HIV/AIDS epidemic exposed the absence of relational rights for non-heterosexuals in a period of accelerating prejudice and growing health needs. Same-sex partners were often marginalized by medical authorities, insurance companies refused cover for same-sex couples, and mortgage companies insisted on HIV tests before agreeing housing loans (Heaphy et al.1999). From the 1980s, the HIV/AIDS epidemic required the building of a community of care-giving, to support those who were suffering and dying from the illness and to offer counselling to their loved ones. This community of care consisted of a tight network of friends, experts and relatives and forced hospitals to relax family-centric visitation policies to include same-sex partners and wider circles of friends (Weston 1991).

The denial of full citizenship to non-heterosexuals also led to child custody disputes, first experienced in the 1970s by lesbian mothers and then extended to fostering and adoption problems experienced by gay and lesbian couples. Controversies involving the care of children confirmed that the term 'family' was much more than just a cosy metaphor applied to non-heterosexual living arrangements. It had legal ramifications and was an essential political tool for the advancement of non-heterosexual politics (Nardi 1999; Weeks et al. 2001). Those who use the term 'families of choice' to describe non-heterosexual relationships generally stress two points: first, the importance of *belonging* and *commitment* to a circle of friends who are seen as corresponding to the familial ideal; and second, the sense of *choice* and *agency* (Weeks et al. 2001:10).

However, a weakness identified in the 'families of choice' approach is a lack of attention to social class. Yvette Taylor (2007) points out that the literature on families of choice tends to abstract class from everyday life and glosses over the constraints and exclusions entailed in many gay and lesbian relationships. Class often disrupts the idealized imaginings of lesbian relationships represented in many studies of the 1990s. Yet social theories such as Giddens' emphasis on the pure relationship and his notion of gay and lesbian couples as a 'vanguard' fail to take account of class. In a study of working-class lesbian life, Taylor (2007) examined issues of sexuality and class using data collected from interviews with fifty-three self-identified working-class lesbians from Scotland and England. She explored the implications of class and sexuality in relation to family, school, work, communities, leisure activities and intimate relationships for lesbian partnerships.

Traditional family values tend to be imposed on gay and lesbian families through these various daily and institutional contexts, according to Taylor. She explains the way city spaces, social scene spaces and everyday spaces are noticeably classed places. She addresses the difficulties faced by working-class lesbian families, such as the negative parental attitudes they face in relation to their children's schooling and choice of residence. The difficulties of class identification are indicated by disagreements between lesbian parents and professionals, such as doctors and teachers, as a feature of the structure of class inexperience. These kinds of negotiations are areas of advantage for confident middle-class parents, whether heterosexual or lesbian. By contrast, working-class lesbian parents sometimes avoid community groups for fear of being perceived and treated negatively. Given that 'good parenting' is often expressed and framed through middle-class norms in social policy, working-class parents are being disadvantaged. They often find it difficult to convey the fact that they are engaged in 'good parenting'(see chapter 3). This problem is amplified for working-class lesbian families. These research examples have thereby identified important issues concerning the intersection of gender, sexuality and class in addressing issues of commitment with regard to the lack of validity of the individualization thesis.

Minority ethnic kinship ties

A further weakness associated with the individualization thesis is a lack of account of the distinctive attributes of minority ethnic families. First, minority ethnic groups are more likely to have *extended kinship* networks than are white European ethnic groups. Second, their family experiences are much more likely to be shaped through processes of settling in an alien culture, known as 'acculturation'. Until recently, much of the literature on families in minority ethnic cultures ignored these features. They revealed the ethnocentric bias towards middle-class white families within family studies (see chapter 1). The extended kinship ties of some minority ethnic families and the matriarchal structure of some single-parent African American and British Caribbean families have either been overlooked by contemporary social theory or interpreted as deviations from a nuclear form. By the 1990s, research tended to concentrate on 'social problems' associated with patterns of discrimination and prejudice against minority ethnic cultures, and their social exclusion. 'Social problems' included housing inequalities, racism and discrimination in the workplace and the community (Goering and Wienk 1997; Modood et al.1997; Bulmer and Solomos 1999; Boal 2000; Mason 2000).

Until recently, studies in both the USA and the UK also focused on the implications for social policy of issues surrounding marital violence, arranged marriages, divorce and single parenthood (see Logan 1996; Toliver 1998). More research in the UK examined the experiences of migration among Black Caribbeans and South Asians by emphasizing the challenges of settling in a new country, exacerbated by discrimination, deprivation, language difficulties, lack of employment opportunities and poor housing as well as separation from family and feelings of isolation or dislocation (Castles and Miller 1998; Koser and Lutz 1998; Chapman 2004). Acculturation is likely to occur over several generations with the offspring, second and third generations gradually finding it easier to fit into the wider, host community.

With regard to extended kinship networks, Black African and Caribbean families generally have more flexible family forms that differ from the nuclear model (Chamberlain 2001). Their extended kinship ties are often characterized by the preservation of strong transnational ties with wider networks valued as a central feature of Caribbean society (Chamberlain 2001; Goulbourne and Chamberlain 2001). Conversely, South Asian families tend to have strictly observed sets of values concerning marriage, with a higher degree of gender segregation in domestic routines than found in most white, Anglophone households (Ghuman 1999; Chapman 2004). In a study of households in what she referred to as a 'Bangladeshi village' in Manchester, Sultana Mustafa Khanum (2001) found that migration played a major role in the formation of households. Many of the men who originated from Bangladesh had two wives and were prohibited by immigration laws from bringing both to the UK. Accordingly, close financial and cultural ties were sustained with kin in Bangladesh, and sometimes political associations too. Khanum (2001) suggests that these relationships impacted on the regulation of their household in the UK, and caused some women, as second wives, to be impoverished and vulnerable. Acculturation is, then, a key factor that influences first-and second-generation minority ethnic migrant families.

Certain minority ethnic families adhere to stricter gender roles, which can restrict women's agency and choices. This suggests that the notion of the 'democratic relationship' portrayed in the individualization thesis is not necessarily a trend or aspiration that characterizes this group. In an ethnographic study of British Pakistani Muslims in Oxford, Alison Shaw (2000) found that young people were internalizing Islamic values and family traditions with intergenerational problems settled largely through negotiation. However, young women experienced specific problems as a result of being treated in more traditional ways than their brothers. This concurs with findings of a study of the relationship between parents and young people in families from different ethnic groups by Brannen et al. (1994), and also research on Sikh girls by Drury (1991).

Generally speaking, minority ethnic families need to be understood in relation to issues of acculturation, biculturalism and religious customs. To conclude, western ideas of individual agency and late modern notions of personhood based on ideas of the 'pure relationship' and the atomized, self-absorbed individual do not necessarily help in understanding contemporary minority ethnic family customs and practices. Thus, sociological analyses of minority ethnic families are now acknowledging distinctive family qualities, such as the likely predominance of extended kin; the likelihood of more rigid gender differences in family roles; differing parenting practices and approaches to ageing and the care of the elderly; distinctive marriage customs that may include arranged marriage (see chapter 6) and divergent approaches and attitudes to fertility (see chapters 7 and 8).

Conclusions

This chapter has drawn attention to the gap between the individualization thesis and concrete evidence in contemporary accounts of changing family life. This problem echoes classic sociological debates of the late nineteenth up to the mid twentieth century, outlined in chapter 1. This chapter has explained that late modern social theorists have identified the development of 'pure relationships', in which new generations of couples abandon traditional family practices and develop autonomous, individualized biographies based on their commitment to one another. The idea of the reflexive agent generated by the individualization thesis has produced a new language of democracy and freedom to explain contemporary forms of intimacy and social relationships. It has also generated a sense of crisis and evoked a fear of decline in long-term commitment in familial relationships. Curiously, the type of family perceived to be declining is not the *extended family* of pre-industrial times but a *modern nuclear* form which has been labelled 'traditional' only recently, since the 1950s (Smart 2007). The disintegration of this newly labelled traditional family unit is indicated by a significant rise in single-headed households, same-sex couples, unmarried cohabiting couples and parents, and post-divorce couples who often bring children into new, 'blended' family relationships. However, the chapter has shown that empirical research findings repeatedly challenge the idea of a decline in family commitment in western nations by highlighting the importance of connectedness among family members (Smart 2007).

'Pure relationships' are not necessarily being fully realized and gender roles are not yet equal. Empirical evidence indicates that Giddens' 'democratic relationship' remains aspirational rather than actual. However, there is also certain evidence that gay and lesbian relationships are forging new ways of practising family as egalitarian relationships, as Giddens argues. As the modern family changes during the early twenty-first century, emotional relations and friendships evolve as new and enduring forms of intimacy that can act as a surrogate family. What we define as 'family' is now more flexible and dynamic, and embraces new kinds of intimacies that were once ignored or condemned.

To conclude, most studies of new, diverse intimate relationships that lie outside marriage and differ from the nuclear norm do not confirm the idea that couples are pursuing relationships of a more democratic but less committed nature. Instead, most findings verify continuities between generations and strong levels of commitment. These issues are revisited in the final chapter of the book in relation to the politics of family values. Meanwhile, the following three chapters examine recent research and debates on personal and family relationships by providing details of the changing patterns and experiences of family life through the lens of parenting, childhood and ageing.

3 Parenting Practices and Values

Parenting is a process embedded in and shaped by wider social values, structures and institutions. Although they may appear natural, the social norms regarding motherhood and fatherhood are socially constructed. This chapter addresses some of the major changes in parenting values and practices from the late twentieth century onwards. It examines parallels and discrepancies between parenting ideals and realities, and the influences of government policy in defining 'parenthood'. The chapter begins by addressing changing meanings and practices of motherhood, including lone motherhood and teenage mothers. This is followed by an enquiry about definitions and the changing status of fatherhood in western societies. Debates about minority ethnic parenting, gay and lesbian parenting issues are examined not only to highlight the diversity of parenting values and practices but also to foreground certain ways in which minority ethnic families have been criticized for diverging from the structures and values of middle-class white families.

Changing ideas about parenthood

Prescriptions for 'good' parenting change over time and across cultures. The period after World War II witnessed increases in women's labour-force participation and the rise in dual-income families in western nations. In the USA and the UK, for example, the earning power of most men fell significantly from the early 1970s, with fewer families able to depend solely on a 'male breadwinner' income. Women entered the workforce in large numbers to contribute to the family income and gain independence. In the USA, 77.5 per cent of working-age women with dependent children now work (United States Bureau of Labor Statistics 2010a). In the UK, more than two-thirds (68 per cent) of working-age women with dependent children are in employment (Office for National Statistics (ONS) 2008b). Although women's widespread movement into paid employment led to questions about who should take responsibility for childcare, many governments have failed to address the childcare needs generated by this trend. This deficit in care is compounded by the rise in lone-parent families, mostly headed by women. When divorce laws were relaxed from the 1970s in most western nations, high rates of marital dissolution occurred alongside other patterns of familial change, including the rise in childbearing outside marriage. The factors of women's employment and rising divorce rates have led to intense public debates about the effects of changing parenting practices on children.

The twentieth-century ideology of egalitarian gender roles in the home and employment has had a major impact on *ideas* about parenting, particularly among women. However, broad trends indicate that, while fathers' participation in their children's lives is increasing, men have not substantially increased their share of domestic chores (Gershuny 2001:198; O'Brien and Shemilt 2003). The gendered division of labour within two-parent households remains surprisingly persistent, with research findings continuing to highlight deep-rooted gendered practices in the allocation of domestic and paid work (Hobson 2002; Craig 2007). Prevailing ideas about men's and women's roles in the home seem to discourage men from performing what is regarded as 'women's work'.

A detailed study of the modern conception of parenting using Australian time-use data by Lyn Craig (2007) found that discrepancies in unpaid work start before the couple have children. She calls this 'the partnership penalty'. When couples form households together, women's unpaid work rises while men's falls, irrespective of the women's motherhood status. The presence of children then intensifies the division of domestic labour. Although marriage is nowadays interpreted as a partnership of two equals, Craig found that the consequences of women's entry into employment contrast with a lack of response from men in terms of balancing their fathering 'responsibilities'. This 'mother penalty' which arises when the couple have children renders women financially worse off across their lifetimes compared to men and child-free women. Referring to the 'dual burden' for women, Craig demonstrates the sheer magnitude of daily hours devoted to children and family by mothers. Her findings confirm previous studies, showing that women are more likely to look after children while undertaking other tasks such as preparing a family meal, and men are more likely to engage in childcare while the mother is also at hand. Of the time fathers spend with their children, a greater proportion is play time and talking to children – something women find difficult to do if they are conducting 'double activities'.

The normative nuclear family is often viewed as a self-sufficient, independent unit and the most effective in raising children. US public policy has therefore focused on strengthening the nuclear family as a major strategy for enhancing the lives of children. Yet half of all households in the USA with young children have two employed parents (Hansen 2005). A key question, then, is whether two-parent families can really be self-sufficient in contemporary western societies. How do working parents provide care and how far do they have to rely on extended networks to support their family needs? In her study of American nuclear families in which both parents were in employment, Karen Hansen found that parents had high work demands and yet also high aspirations to be intensely involved in their children's lives. These two sets of demands combined to make parents feel overwhelmed, generating a great deal of parental anxiety. Hansen points out that this is a *structural* conflict, caused by ineffective work/life balance policies. Yet parents experienced the tension as *personal* problems. She found that parents' capacities to care for their children were helped or hindered by the availability or lack of an informal network of kin or friends, a reciprocating network that could be called upon to help.

Hansen found class differences, with working-class and middle-class American families relying more on their wider kin for help, while professional middle classes and upper classes relied more on friends and paid help. The loose, weak ties typical of upper-and middle-class professional couples may be useful for networking for job resources. However, they appear to be ineffective in mobilizing resources for rearing children on a daily basis. The creation of strong, personalized and kinship ties were the most effective for working families. These kinds of ties were found among working-class and middle-class families. Nevertheless, well-resourced upper-class families were able to overcome any deficiencies in the quality of networks by paying for care. Hansen exposes the myth that families in the USA are independent, isolated and self-reliant units. She found that mothers, in particular, have to navigate this ideology of parenting in relation to their dependence on others for help.

Morality and motherhood

This ideology of parenting relates to the question of the 'morality' of parenting practices. The principles that govern notions of 'good' motherhood can differ significantly according to families' class and ethnic backgrounds. In western societies today, the morality of the mother's behaviour is generally gauged by socially acceptable norms about 'proper' family life which, in turn, continue to be shaped by a nuclear family ideal. Research indicates that mothers tend to see their own motherhood role in relation to these wider social norms (Ribbens McCarthy et al. 2000; May 2008). Confirming Hansen's argument of the impossibility of independence for modern families, research indicates an increasing gap between the way mothering is perceived and how it is practised (Maher and Saugeres 2007). This corresponds with the mothering challenges brought about by divorce, separation and lone parenthood.

Several recent studies indicate that mothers articulate a strong moral imperative of putting their children's needs first (Smart and Neale 1999; Ribbens McCarthy et al. 2000, 2003). However, there are significant differences in the ways that 'good' motherhood and 'good' fatherhood are socially constructed and perceived. The ethic of care for children is paramount for mothers. The mother is perceived as the core of the family, as its emotional stabilizer that keeps the whole family together (Vuori 2001; Ribbens McCarthy et al. 2003). Indeed, the role of 'good' motherhood appears to include responsibility for the quality of fatherhood: a 'good' mother ensures that her children receive 'good' fathering. Bad fathering is frequently blamed on the mother (May 2003). Often, the implication is that 'absent fatherhood' is somehow the fault of the mother.

A key problem is that divorce, cohabitation and lone parenthood are still viewed within dominant public discourses as signs of moral decline, despite being widespread. Divorce rates have steadily risen since the mid-1970s when divorce laws eased the process of legally ending a marriage. Over a third of marriages now end in divorce in western countries. For example, UK divorce rates indicate that approximately 45 per cent of marriages will end in divorce (ONS 2008a), while in the USA, the rate is slightly lower at 40 per cent

(United States Census B   '010b). The majority of lone-parent families are headed by women (for example, 80–90 per cent in Europe (Lehmann and Wirtz 2004)). The largest group of lone mothers is comprised of those who have experienced a marital breakdown, followed by widows. The smallest category consists of lone mothers who have never married, although this group is rising in relation to temporary as well as long-term cohabitation. Evidence also suggests that women from working-class backgrounds are more likely than middle-class women to become lone mothers, especially never-married lone mothers (Kiernan et al. 1998).

A range of research indicates that divorce is harmful to children. Findings are often used to argue that divorce is morally indefensible. Lone mothers frequently experience prejudice, stigma and personal doubts over their ability to bring their children up 'properly' (Roseneil and Mann 1996; May 2001). Research on media representations in the USA and UK demonstrate that lone parents are often defined, particularly by the tabloid press, as 'undeserving scroungers' (Atkinson et al. 1998; Wright and Jagger 1999; Chambers 2001). The 'demoralization' perspective – that divorce leads to bad parenting – is supported by a well-known 1980 study of sixty American families after divorce, by Wallerstein and Kelly (1980). Their findings showed that children suffer socially, emotionally and educationally from divorce and repeat the pattern of divorce in their own marriages. Research in the 1990s also suggested that children in families headed by lone mothers are disadvantaged by the lack of a father figure, that they are exposed to poverty and even bad parenting (Cockett and Tripp 1994). More recent findings indicate that children from lone-parent families are more likely to experience poverty or reduced economic circumstances compared to those who live in two-parent families (Rainwater and Smeeding 2003; Fischer 2007; McLanahan 2007). For instance, in 2007/8, 91 per cent of lone parents with dependent children and 56 per cent of couples with dependent children received income-related benefits in the UK (ONS 2010). In response to such findings, successive governments in the USA and UK have called for a strengthening of family values, arguing that all children should be able to grow up in a stable nuclear family comprised of a heterosexual, married couple (see Fox Harding 1999; Wright and Jagger 1999; and chapter 9).

However, the risk of economic hardship differs by country, demonstrating the role of a range of social and economic factors. These factors include major national differences in government support for lone-parent families; differences in financial contributions from fathers; and the differences in educational levels and individual profiles of the lone parents themselves. In Nordic countries, for example, children in lone-parent families are less likely to be impoverished than in the UK or Ireland due to effective state support and the higher levels of educational and employment achievements of their mothers (Kiernan et al. 2007). In an important Finnish study by Vanessa May (2008), a major difference in circumstances was found between older and younger generations of lone mothers. Older lone mothers who had lower living standards in the mainly agrarian society of post-World War II Finland found it difficult to provide the basic necessities or education that their children needed to advance in life. Lone mothers therefore prioritized basic necessities. By contrast, younger generations of lone mothers prioritized their children's emotional and psychological well-being rather than basic necessities. For this younger group, Finland had become an affluent post-industrial society with an effective welfare state and a high standard of living. Younger lone mothers tended to be relatively well-educated middle-class career women, which influences the lack of hardship in their life stories. Divorce has become more acceptable and lone motherhood is less stigmatized there. Nevertheless, the younger lone mothers were in agreement that children fare better in two-parent families, indicating the strength of nuclear-family ideology.

The public condemnation of single-mother welfare recipients, as evidence of the moral breakdown of society, deeply affects how the single mothers see their roles as parent (see Stacey 1994). A study of single, working-class mothers in a small town in the US state of Vermont by Margaret Nelson (2002, 2005) found that the women were aware of the negative perception of single-mother welfare recipients as lazy, unmotivated, likely to cheat, and as having children simply to increase their benefits. These single, mainly white women were very concerned about how they were viewed by others, including family and friends, their welfare officers and the public at large. However, the study also found that the single mothers justified their reliance on state assistance by sustaining a belief in their own self-worth. They differentiated themselves from other welfare recipients and expressed values of self-sufficiency. In their attempts to resist shame, they were proud that they did not have to rely on friends and family, and felt they were performing an important role in bringing up their children.

Social class and ethnic identity are significant factors for lone mothers and their children (Rowlingson and McKay 2005). Middle-class lone mothers have better resources and opportunities. They remain lone mothers for less time and may have little in common with a young single mother who has few resources and bleak prospects. In her study of motherhood by choice, Rosanna Hertz (2006) shows that having children outside of marriage is a fast-growing phenomenon among mainly middle-class women who have the resources to be successful single mothers. She estimates that approximately 2.7 million American women are single mothers by choice. Through interviews with 65 women, with 17 per cent being lesbian or bisexual women, Hertz documented how middle-class women have managed to make single parenthood work for them. Hertz discovered that many of the women believed in marriage (or committed partnerships), particularly as a context for childbearing, but they had reached a critical point at which they perceived it to be unattainable in their own lives. Marriage was endorsed as an ideal by many of the heterosexual women, but was often seen to have little relevance to real life. For these mothers, their attachment to career and the sense of independence associated with it, prompted them to take a different route from that of a traditional marriage with children. Once they had become mothers, they struggled to conform to the conventional definitions of motherhood. Broader cultural tensions around marriage and childbearing are, then, raised by such a study.

Hertz found that deciding to have a baby outside of a heterosexual partnership involves complicated steps and choices. Nearly all the methods involved contractual agreements that clarify the rights of the parties involved. Some approached a sperm donor bank and rebuilt a 'father profile' when the child was born. Some attempted pregnancy with an uncertain romantic partner and had to address those legal implications. Others created a transracial family through adoption or a 'transacting family' involving committed gay partners. Despite using the unconventional methods of IVF or adoption to become mothers, these women conformed to conventional rules about child-rearing. Challenging questions are raised about the future role of fathers in a society where not only has sex been uncoupled from marriage but also childbearing has become separated from marriage and from fatherhood.

Certain countries, including France, Denmark, Sweden and Australia, treat lone-parent families in the same way as other single-income families. Since 'lone mothers' are such a diverse group in terms of social class, gender, ethnicity and nation, Rowlingson and McKay (2005) argue that the very concept of 'lone mother' needs to be reconsidered in terms of its legitimacy as an analytical device. They state: 'The value of putting these different types of women into a single analytical category seems questionable both in social policy terms and in broader sociological terms' (2005:47). A simplistic focus on family structure may therefore need to be questioned, particularly when we examine these issues cross-nationally (Millar 2001).

Teenage mothers

In contrast to the 'mothers by choice' studied by Hertz, teenage mothers tend to come from lower-income families. Teenage pregnancies have declined in western nations since the late 1960s and early 1970s. Yet they remain persistently high in the UK, USA, New Zealand and Canada, compared to continental Europe (UNICEF 2003). Teenage pregnancies have, like single-parent families, traditionally carried a social stigma. During the 1950s and 1960s, most teenage parents were pressured into marriage as a common 'remedy' to avoid the shame associated with illegitimacy. About 20 per cent of the offspring were adopted soon after their birth. By 2000, the majority of teenage parents remained unmarried. However, around half cohabited with the father, and another quarter jointly registered the birth with the father, indicating a continuing parental relationship (Selman, 1996, 2003). The shift away from marriage towards unmarried cohabitation and 'living apart together' are changes matched by wider trends for the population as a whole (Barlow et al. 2005; Haskey 2005).

In the USA and UK, the public dialogue about teenage parenting forms part of the discourse about moral decline associated with marriage, single parenting and teenage sexuality (Duncan and Edwards 1999; Selman 2003; Williams 2004; Wilson and Huntington 2005). However, teenage motherhood is regarded differently among different social groups. For example, if a teenage daughter becomes pregnant among British middle-class families, an abortion is usually arranged to prevent her from being disadvantaged in terms of her future life-course options (ONS 2000; Chambers et al. 2004b). Younger women in poorer neighbourhoods are more liable to become pregnant, and least likely to consider abortion as an option for dealing with an unplanned pregnancy. Among certain working-class communities, there is less or no stigma associated with teenage motherhood, and the daughter may be provided with wider kin support in caring for the child (Seamark and Lings 2004).

Government policies in the USA and UK have reflected public discourses of disapproval. For instance, British government strategies have approached teenage parents as casualties of misinformation, ignorance and low aspirations. This is exemplified by the framework for policy in the Social Exclusion Unit (SEU 1999) report. The report states that pregnancy is viewed as a solution by girls who have no employment prospects and that many teenagers are ignorant of the facts about contraception, sexually transmitted infections, relationships and parenthood. The SEU report states that these factors correspond with social disadvantage. Yet current policy views tend to stress *individual* behaviour and motivations, rather than the wider *structural* influences on behaviour associated with poverty and other forms of related social disadvantage (Arai 2003:203).

At a global level, the influential UNICEF report 'Teenage Births in Rich Nations' claims that teenage mothers are:

> much more likely to drop out of school, to have low or no qualifications, to be unemployed or low paid, to grow up without a father, to become a victim of neglect and abuse, to do less well at school, to become involved in crime, use drugs and alcohol. (UNICEF 2003:3)

However, Simon Duncan (2007) points out that the statistical methodology used by UNICEF is flawed. Teenage mothers are being compared with *all* mothers rather than those of a similar age and social background. He argues that becoming a young mother may not be the cause of the poor outcomes regarding education, employment and income. Rather, both young motherhood and poor outcomes may be caused by social disadvantages experienced before pregnancy. Most research on teen parenthood is quantitative and therefore fails to identify teen parents' qualitative experiences of parenting in terms of social class, ethnic identity and community/region. Quantitative research can be beneficial in identifying broad patterns and trends, but tends to approach teen parents as a static, unchanging group. Duncan (2007:329) also argues that policy may be better directed at improving employment for young people as a whole in declining labour markets, and regenerating disadvantaged neighbourhoods, rather than simply at targeting teen parenting in itself.

Traditional and new models of fatherhood

With rising expectations about romance, intimacy and family life, traditional models of fatherhood are progressively being called into question by female partners and by a range of social institutions. The responsibilities and practices associated with fatherhood are not as clear-cut or as morally regulated as those of motherhood (Miller 2010). Nevertheless, dominant discourses of 'good' fatherhood are apparent. Until recently, the concepts of the 'male breadwinner' or father as 'family provider' have been linked with familial legitimacy in western societies. Indeed, within family-values rhetoric, ideas about absent fatherhood are often founded on the traditional breadwinner role (Townsend 2002). In order for the state to avoid the burden of family welfare, the father must provide financial support and be reaffirmed as the 'head' of the family. The absence of fatherhood in households headed by women as an outcome of divorce, separation, teenage pregnancies or lesbian partnerships is perceived by many politicians to be undermining the traditional concept of 'the family' (see chapter 9).

Recent studies chart the ways in which fatherhood is being reshaped against the backdrop of changing policies about the role of fatherhood after divorce, changing modes of heterosexual masculinity and patterns of male employment (Townsend 2002; O'Brien and Shemilt 2003; Brannen and Nilsen 2006; Williams 2008). Models of fathering indicate a shift from traditional 'breadwinner' as an unemotional disciplinarian to the much celebrated father as 'new man'. As mentioned, recent changes in western labour markets have made it difficult for men to sustain the traditional fathering role of male breadwinner (Townsend 2002). Well-paid jobs, long-term employment and the conventional gendered division of labour within the family, which once shaped the father's role in the family, have gradually been eroded. Yet research shows that fathers often identify with the ideal type of financial provider (Warin et al. 1999; O'Brien and Shelmit 2003; Williams 2008). Today, 'good' fathers are assessed on the extent of their *involvement* with children as well as the performance of other responsibilities such as moral and educational teacher, sex-role model and provider (Lamb 1995).

The emphasis nowadays is on a more 'involved' role for fathers, from policy-makers and female partners. However, the notion of 'new man' used to indicate an emergent and more involved form of fatherhood has been criticized for being more of an aspiration than a reality (LaRossa 1988). Many scholars agree that there has been little alteration in fathers' contributions to family life and deny the notion of a changing fathering role. Yet this depends largely on how 'contribution' is defined. Esther Dermott's (2008) research concurs that fatherhood has changed to encompass emotions and the expression of affection. However, she also argues that it does not amount to sharing equally in childcare with mothers. There may be little evidence of men's increased contribution to housework but there is emerging evidence that men spend more time with their children than in the past. There is also growing evidence that, in households where both parents are employed, men are taking more responsibility for childcare even though both men and women identify the mother as the main carer (O'Brien and Shemilt 2003). Evidence suggests that fathers aspire to do more with their children (Henwood and Proctor 2003).

While British and US government policy attempts to *involve* fathers directly in parenting, the concept of provider is still being promoted in policy discourse, leading to some ambiguity in terms of the signals being sent to parents. For example, under the recent Labour government of 1997–2009 in the UK, fatherhood was presented in a framework that emphasized that men must be responsible for the *financial* provision for their families and themselves (Williams 2008:495). This approach contrasts with the idea of 'involvement' in parenting relationships that fosters equality between parents. The 'provider' for the family is the central principle behind an old-style fathering identity, and this is leaving men confused in their interpretation of the new fathering role (Chadwick and Heffernan 2003; Williams 2008). An American study by Nicholas Townsend (2002) about men's changing views and experiences of fatherhood, confirmed that fatherhood is composed of four elements: emotional closeness, provision, protection and endowment. However, Townsend discovered that fathers still viewed the traditional provider role as paramount:

> Of these four, men said the most important thing they did for their children was to provide for them. This identification of fatherhood and providing is crucial, reflecting the central place of employment in men's sense of self-worth and helping to explain many of the apparent anomalies in men's accounts. (285)

While government policies in the USA and UK have been emphasizing the father's role as a financial provider since the late 1990s, they have also been promoting a policy of advising practitioners in schools, health care and children's centres to 'engage' fathers (Featherstone 2010). The promotion of father involvement with children is assumed to produce good outcomes, especially for disadvantaged children. However, feminist scholars point out that mothers' poor pay and gendered inequalities in the workforce tend to be ignored (Lister 2006; Lewis and Campbell 2007). Moreover, by constructing the father–child relationship as dyadic, the role that mothers have played historically in facilitating men's fathering role gets obscured (Featherstone 2010). The US and UK policy focus on engaging fathers contrasts with policy on parenting in continental Europe and the Nordic countries. Governments in many Nordic countries have introduced more comprehensive changes at policy level which give men and women *universal* entitlements to balance work and care, through comprehensive childcare support and paternity leave entitlement. These rights are provided as part of a commitment to promoting citizenship rights that acknowledge gendered disparities (see Lister 2009).

A key issue, here, is the amount of support given by the state to fathers as well as mothers, to make use of parental leave and to be involved in childcare. Lewis and Campbell (2007) have summarized the considerable evidence from cross-national research on the kind of effective parental leave that fathers would be likely to take: it must be an individual entitlement, paid at a high rate of compensation, and be flexible, making possible shorter and longer blocks of leave either full-or part-time. Parental leave arrangements in the Nordic welfare states have enabled *both* parents to look after very young children at home. Sweden, Iceland and Denmark have been classified as key examples of a 'one-year-leave gender equality orientated model', and Finland and Norway are examples of a 'parental choice orientated model' which also places (less explicit) emphasis on gender equality (Lister 2009:254). Ruth Lister argues that this is of particular significance for gendered citizenship. She asserts that governments need to recognize that men's and women's access to citizenship rights and ability to act as citizens in the public sphere are differentially affected by their responsibilities in the private sphere of the family. Despite the UK government's desire to 'involve' fathers in parenting, the range of policies concerning the balancing of work and care has a limited focus on fathers. For example, UK paternity leave lags behind maternity leave. Paternity leave of up to two weeks has been introduced, paid at a flat rate (which is relatively low) and not earnings related. Mothers receive six weeks' maternity leave paid at 90 per cent of their earnings, and 29 or 30 weeks paid at lower, income-support levels, totalling nine months.

Fatherhood after divorce

A so-called 'crisis of fatherhood' after divorce has prompted a reconstruction of fatherhood in law and social policy in the UK and USA (Smart and Neale 1999; Collier 2005; Collier and Sheldon 2008). In their review of families with young children in the USA, Demos and Cox (2000) found that more than a quarter of divorced fathers had not seen their children at all in the previous year; only 27 per cent saw them at least weekly; and less than a third of children had the opportunity to spend extended periods of time with fathers. More than half of the fathers were not involved in their children's lives and just under half had paid any child maintenance in the previous year. Those fathers who were more involved with their children post-divorce tended to have been closer to them prior to divorce, to live near their children and to have joint custody. In western nations, there is a new emphasis on the centrality of the father, within a new pro-contact paradigm in post-divorce family life (Collier and Sheldon 2008). The now dominant pro-contact philosophy in UK law contrasts with earlier beliefs that a 'clean break' was best for couples after divorce, with fathers not automatically allowed to see their children. Paternal contact with the child is increasingly viewed not only as a child's right but also as essential to children's welfare, even though the evidence for the latter remains vague.

A number of groups, including politicians and governments, men's organizations and charities, have argued for fathers to take on a more central role in families after divorce by developing strategies to encourage enduring commitment from fathers in relationships with their children. However, campaigners on domestic violence continue to express considerable concern about the implications of the new pro-contact emphasis and about the low levels of court refusal of contact given the prevalence of domestic violence (Harrison 2008). Others note that mothers may be obliged to continue with an inequitable gendered division of labour after divorce – even if that was precisely the problem that they sought to end through divorce (Reece 2006). Mothers run the risk of being considered obstructive if they raise concerns about men's reliability or poor parenting (Wallbank 2007). The amount of practical and emotional work mothers may need to undertake to ensure that father contact is beneficial to children has been obscured within policy and legislative developments (Featherstone 2010).

The difficulty here, then, is that the term 'involvement' is ambiguous and ill-defined. As Brid Featherstone points out, the concept is usually not specified in policy documents:

> It is never suggested, for example, that it might be sharing in childcare, making medical appointments and so on. Whilst such suggestions on the part of the state would raise legitimate worries about how such measures might be enforced and the author is very sceptical about any such project, it is possible to see the agenda as accepting an inequitable gendered division of labour. (2010:215)

However, while the discourse of the 'involved father' in Britain and the USA is more ambiguous, it is commonplace in Scandinavian countries (Brandth and Kvande 2003). In order to be sensitive to the challenges of today's changing fathering practices, it is important to learn more about policy in other nations: for example, about how resident fathers interact with their children and about the difficulties faced by both post-divorce partners in addressing pro-contact policy.

Minority ethnic parenting

The parenting practices of minority ethnic parents in countries such as the USA and UK have been so poorly researched and understood that they require separate attention here. Despite a surge in interest in families and parenting by policy-makers and researchers, recent reviews also demonstrate a narrow knowledge of parenting among minority, or 'minoritized', ethnic populations in the UK (Allgar et al. 2003; Phoenix and Husain 2007). Earlier research into minority ethnic parenting in the 1970s was criticized for being framed by ethnocentric principles and for failing to deal with issues that are of greatest concern to minority parents themselves (Pollack 1979). Research can often serve to perpetuate stereotypes by treating particular minority groups as homogeneous rather than diverse (Modood et al. 1997). In the USA and UK, African American, Black and South Asian parents have been subjected to particular scrutiny due to persistent anxieties about their parenting practices.

Early reports in the USA highlight themes about minority ethnic parenting that became standard in both Britain and the USA. Governments and academics were concerned with poor educational and employment outcomes for African American and British African Caribbean children, and also Hispanic and other minority ethnic children in the USA. Studies such as the Swann report in the UK typically assessed these poor outcomes in relation to differences from white majority ethnic families in terms of family composition and household arrangements, parenting styles and disciplinary routines (Department of Education and Science 1985). Simplistic and essentialist ideas about parents of American African and British African Caribbean origin have tended to dominate debates, based on assumptions that they cannot control their children and make inadequate parents (e.g. Phoenix 1996; Small 2002). More recent research on families and ethnicity continues to exhibit problems. Distinctions in minority ethnic parenting and children's outcomes are often interpreted as shortcomings or deviations from a white nuclear-family norm (Phoenix and Husain 2007). Studies of 'parenting' tend to focus excessively on mothers. Fathers are usually highlighted when father absence is being studied.

Research in the USA suggests, then, that African American, Asian American and Latino parents have parenting styles that differ from those observed and standardized among white, European American, middle-class parents (Roschelle 1997). There is, however, no clear consensus on exactly how they differ or how they relate to child and adolescent outcomes. This is partly because research is limited and often less methodologically precise than studies of parenting among white European Americans (McLoyd et al. 2000). British research has found that cultural practices are not transferred simply from parents' countries of origin to Britain or from parents to children, but are specific to the socio-economic context in which they arise (Kotchick and Forehand 2002). For example, the tendency for Black British mothers to be employed when they have children results not just from both historical and cultural factors but also from high rates of unemployment for Black men and low rates of pay for both Black men and Black women (Reynolds 2001). A study of parents among minority ethnic families in the UK by Ravinder Barn (Barn, with Ladino and Rogers 2006) found that low income, unemployment and poor housing were characteristic of Black, Pakistani and Bangladeshi families. A lack of financial resources, coupled with poor and overcrowded housing, led to very difficult situations for some parents. Many of the Caribbean families experiencing financial and housing problems were lone mothers. Among all minority ethnic groups, the wider family was a strong source of support for many parents, who described contact with relatives as an important ingredient in the upbringing of their children (Barn 2006).

Minority ethnic fathers have received remarkably little research attention (Lewis and Lamb 2007). Studies indicate a preoccupation with the effects of 'father absence' on children, with particular reference to African American and African Caribbean fathers (Phoenix and Husain 2007). However, the common view that fathers are 'absent' from their children's lives if they are non-resident has been challenged. For example, in the USA, King and colleagues (2004) found that white adolescents had higher contact levels with non-resident fathers than African American or Hispanic young people. After controlling for socio-economic status, they found that variations between ethnic groups were further reduced. In general, the higher the level of fathers' education and income, the more likely they were to be involved with their non-resident children (King et al. 2004). In a study of British Black families, Tracey Reynolds (2005) found that non-resident fathers contributed to their children's lives in a variety of ways.

In an exploration of fathering behaviours and experiences among British Asian men, Salway et al. (2009) studied four religio-ethnic Asian 'groups' – Bangladeshi Muslims, Pakistani Muslims, Gujarati Hindus and Punjabi Sikhs. Their findings highlight the great family diversity that exists within ethnic 'groups'. Across all groups, becoming a father was approached as a significant life stage and a key element of self-identity for the majority of fathers. For many, having children was considered to be an element of the *extended family*, beyond the husband–wife couple. Fatherhood corresponded with responsibility, commitment and self-esteem. Demonstrating the persistence of the 'breadwinner' model, income-earning was persistently viewed as a fundamental aspect of being a father. Research by Hauari and Hollingworth (2009) on fathering, masculinity and diversity in England among Pakistani, white British, Black Caribbean and Black African families found that economic provision continued to define the father's role and conceptions of 'good fathering', reflecting views associated with white fathering. Regardless of ethnic group, all of the fathers shared challenges in their role as parents. The difficulties they experienced were mainly due to practical situations, including work commitments, long working hours, unemployment or poor health. These findings support policy recommendations that promote a better work/life balance for fathers, increased financial support for families on low incomes and increased parenting support for fathers.

Gay and lesbian parenting

The new patterns of intimacy being created by gay and lesbian families, and claims to relational rights, are contesting traditional conceptions of family and parenting (Weeks et al. 2001:2). Before the gay liberation era of the 1960s and 1970s, the cultural perception of the family as intrinsically heterosexual was so widely acknowledged as to be almost incontrovertible. In 1960s America, lesbian mothers and gay fathers who came out in the process of a divorce from husbands and wives frequently faced the threat of losing custody of their children and even contact with them. Custody case proceedings from the late 1960s to the mid-1980s reveal strong state investment in preserving the family as a *heterosexual* institution. This investment was supported by official conceptions of the 'homosexual'. It was assumed that a gay man or lesbian was more likely to abuse or somehow transmit their sexual orientation to their children, and that the children of lesbians and gay men would be encumbered by social stigma.

By constructing same-sex sexuality as antithetical to parenting, this institutionalized prejudice actively removed parental rights from many lesbians and gay men. A whole generation of lesbian and gay parents experienced the dread of being separated from their children. For example, by 1985 an increasing number of state courts in the USA overturned decisions that denied lesbian mothers and gay fathers custody and visitation rights. These early years of custody cases demonstrate the powerful cultural link between sexual orientation and the family and the slow and challenging changes that took place. Lesbians and gay men had to battle to transform widespread beliefs that parenting is exclusively heterosexual, and the legal practices that reinforced this view (Rivers 2010). Between 1967 and 1985, most American custody cases concerned men and women who had left heterosexual marriages.

Gay fathers generally argued for visitation rights, and lesbians contested for visitation or custody. Lesbians and gay men who contested these practices in court formed part of a wider resistance movement that opposed heterosexist, racist and misogynistic attitudes towards the organization of the 'normal' American family. After 1985, the modern lesbian, gay, bisexual and transsexual (LGBT) freedom struggle gradually prioritized family and domestic rights, which became the central issues of the movement by the end of the twentieth century (Rivers 2010:936). In most US jurisdictions today, lesbianism is no longer taken into account in custody proceedings. However, gay male parents continue to be rendered problematic, partly because mothers more commonly preserve custody of children after divorce and stereotypes prevail about gay men as fathers.

In the 1970s and 1980s, activists campaigned to revise attitudes towards gay and lesbian parenting and relied on professional support (see, for example, Goodman 1977; Green 1992). Such studies contributed to changes in legal attitudes towards lesbian and gay parents during the period. Through the 1980s, the standard argument by psychologists sympathetic to lesbian and gay parents was that lesbians and gay men raised children who did not differ in any significant way from those raised in single-parent heterosexual households. Research into these emergent family structures demonstrates that heterosexual parenting is not necessary for children to thrive. Numerous research studies have been reviewed that examined many areas of family life, including psychological adjustment, self-esteem, sexual abuse, bullying in schools, social relationships and academic performance (see Stacey and Biblarz 2001; Goldberg 2010). These studies demonstrate that children of lesbian parents do not show any signs of psychological problems (Dunne 1999; Johnson and O'Connor 2002; Golombok et al. 2003; Gartrell et al. 2005; Gartrell and Bos 2010). This body of research has been instrumental in changing laws to support same-sex parents in custody battles and adoption decisions. Much research on GLBT families draws attention to the heterosexist norms that surround the nuclear family (Riggs 2007).

The diversity of gay and lesbian families makes them difficult to define. Indeed, the gay and lesbian 'family' is a contested concept (Weston 1991). Although most children of same-sex parents come from former heterosexual relations, a growing number of children are planned and born into a homosexual context. Lesbian women who plan to have children face the practical challenge of finding a 'father'. They also need to consider whether they wish to engage in a life-long commitment with the biological 'father'. The child may have a 'known father' or an 'anonymous sperm donor'. If the 'father' is known, the question is whether he should participate in the care of the child or not and whether he should be a known father with shared custody or without shared custody (Folgerø 2008; Ryan-Flood 2009). Having children in a homosexual family challenges cultural understandings of what is 'natural' (Folgerø 2008). Biological ideas about gender, sexuality, kinship, childhood and parenthood continue to influence the public debate on lesbian and gay adoptive rights. Because same-sex partners must involve a third person in order to have a child, the child will have a biological link to that person. How lesbian mothers and gay fathers think about and cope with their own family practices in relation to these hegemonic norms are being explored in contemporary research (see Ryan-Flood 2009).

By reconfiguring family, kinship, relationships, parenthood and reproduction, these 'new family' practices have the subversive poten-tial of fracturing and destabilizing of the hetero/homo binary (Weeks et al. 1999a). They confirm the constructed nature of heterosexual relationships (Butler 1999 [1990]:86). Although GLBT parenthood challenges apparently fixed categories such as 'father' and 'mother', evidence indicates that lesbian mothers' and gay fathers' own accounts are often ambiguous and that they redefine their own family practices in a range of ways. They may simultaneously transgress and yet reproduce heteronormative assumptions about childhood, father-hood, motherhood, family and kinship (Folgerø 2008). For same-sex couples, the inclusion of children can be a *display* of familyness (Finch 2007).

The most notable advances in new scholarship on lesbian, gay, bisexual and transgender families in the past decade have been about planned lesbian co-mother families. Cumulative evidence suggests that many such families have comparatively high levels of shared labour and parental investment, yet they may not be as 'genderless' as previously portrayed (see chapter 2). Whether gay or lesbian couples have children from a previous relationship or decide to have children through a donor, it is likely that one partner will give up career pros-pects to concentrate on parenting. In these circumstances, similar problems arise to those identified above in heterosexual family relationships (Biblarz and Savci 2010).

Conclusions

This chapter has explained that dramatic changes in family life have generated anxieties among US and British governments about

parenting practices. Parenting policies tend to be framed by traditional family values in efforts to standardize parenting practices in the
context of divorce and lone parenting. In particular, the strong moral
framework shaping views on motherhood and the notion of 'involved'
fatherhood motivates much state policy. US and British parenting
policies differ considerably from those in other parts of Europe, particularly Nordic countries. Motherhood has traditionally been highly
regulated by public ideals about and policies on 'good motherhood' in
the USA and UK. Yet motherhood is increasingly being experienced
as a role *outside* conventional marriage. The drive towards 'democratic', 'pure relationships' has led to higher expectations among
women about the sharing of parenting. However, gender stereotypes
of parental roles prevail in family life, with women continuing to find
themselves burdened by high domestic and childcare loads before
and after divorce.

Importantly, fatherhood is transforming and governments
are increasingly motivated to regulate this role. This chapter has
shown that fatherhood is gradually moving from a traditional one-
dimensional role to a more multi-dimensional one, with expectations
that a father should be involved in all aspects of childcare and childrearing activities. Nevertheless, the model of the male breadwinner /
female homemaker continues to have a powerful influence on parental attitudes and policy. The rise in divorce and teen parenthood fuel
concerns that fatherhood is being marginalized and should become a
more central presence. Defining and supporting 'fathering' is high on
the political agenda for British and US policy-makers. Governments
are promoting the idea of more 'involvement' by fathers, yet also
wanting fathers to sustain an outdated breadwinner role. Learning
more about how resident and non-resident fathers interact with their
children, finding out about the difficulties faced by both post-divorce
partners in addressing pro-contact policy, and studying policy objectives and outcomes in other nations are all important requirements
for policy-makers to help parents meet the challenges of today's
changing parenting practices.

This chapter has also emphasized that the parenting practices of
minority ethnic groups are diverse rather than homogeneous. Yet
our understanding of minority ethnic families in the UK and USA
has been hampered by ethnocentric research methodologies in which
minority ethnic families have been compared unfavourably with
white, nuclear-family practices. More recent sensitive and in-depth

research reveals the importance of understanding minority ethnic family life in the context of migration, ethnicity, identity and belonging and also by taking into account the political, social and economic climate as well as processes of 'otherness' in the host society. Chapter 6 expands on some of the issues raised here about transnational family and kinship networks. It places debates about family formation and family arrangements in the global context of marriage and migration.

The parenting practices of GLBT families have led the way in challenging many time-honoured conventions about parenting. As we have seen, legal attitudes towards gay and lesbian parenting have changed since the 1980s in western nations such as the USA and UK, as a result of major studies showing that children can thrive when brought up by gay and lesbian parents as well as in heterosexual families. Research has also highlighted the concept of the 'new family', discussed in chapter 2, in which GBLT parenthood subverts heteronormative assumptions about parenthood. The following chapter explores changing ideas about childhood agency and family life, and shows how they have impacted on children's experiences and parent–child relationships in relation to pressures associated with new media use in the home and the commercialization and privatization of children's lives.

4 The Changing Nature of Childhood

As the previous chapter explains, the rise of post-divorce parenting and single parenthood are prompting government and public anxieties about parental roles and relationships with children. A key shift has also taken place in public attitudes to childhood which impact dramatically on parenting and childhood. Nowadays, child-rearing in western cultures is characterized less by the authoritarian parenting associated with past traditional societies and more by a *negotiation* between parent and child in a process monitored by the state and other agencies such as schools and welfare organizations. An *emotional investment* in children is typically viewed as the dominant approach to 21st-century childhood in public discourses about the family. Yet contemporary ideas about children are shaped by a tension between two opposing accounts of childhood: *children as agents in their own right* with choices about how to live their lives and *children as innocent* and in need of protection. Upheld by the United Nations Convention on the Rights of the Child of 1989,[1] today's children have enhanced rights, first in the form of a right to a childhood, and then as a right to be treated more like adults with access to certain privileges of the adult world. This rights framework has coincided with a significant change in the balance of power in families, between parents and children. Yet the idea of *childhood agency*, in which the child is recognized as a person with rights, conflicts with the *romantic ideal* that children are innocent and vulnerable and have a right to be childlike. The practicalities of contemporary childrearing practices are set against this romantic ideal and rights discourse, often leading to confusion for both parents and children.

This chapter examines the effects of key trends and processes on children's lives. These trends include rising divorce rates; state interventions in response to divorce and other changes in family life; the growing emphases on consumption in children's lives; the accelerated use of new media in the home; and the growing privatization of childhood. The experiences of contemporary childhood have changed dramatically in the last three generations. First, the rise in divorce rates and in diverse family forms is leading to new kinds of connections between parents and children, as the previous chapter shows. Second, children across the globe have had accelerated contact with commercialism, the media and new technologies in the second half of the twentieth century (Zelizer 1985; Cunningham 1995; Buckingham 2007). These sorts of exposure highlight the tension between childhood agency and the parental need and compulsion to protect children from the risks associated with consumerism and accelerated new media communication. The issues here are explored in relation to an assessment of recent theories of childhood and empirical studies of experiences of childhood in western and developing countries.

Past ideas about childhood

Debate about whether or not 'childhood' is an invention of the modern period began with the work of Philippe Ariès (1962). He argued that the idea of childhood as 'a distinct phase in the life course' was absent in the European Middle Ages. Instead, children were treated like small adults and absorbed into the routines of the family household and working life, with no particular protection or rights. Ariès drew his conclusions largely from studying representations of children in medieval portraiture. He found that children were portrayed wearing the same styles of clothing as adults. They lacked the stylized depictions of innocence, charm and vulnerability such as large eyes and chubby features with which we are familiar today in visual images of childhood. However, Ariès has been criticized for speculating from limited sources (Vann 1982; Pollock 1983). Portrait paintings were highly stylized and confined to a small wealthy elite group whose attitudes towards children may not have represented the views of wider society. Nevertheless, his main assertion, that the separateness of the status and identity of childhood is a social construction of the modern period, is generally accepted by social scientists.

A major influence on today's ideas about childhood in Europe has been a shift from valuing children for their economic worth to valuing them for emotional reasons (Zelizer 1985; Cunningham

1995). Historical studies in the USA indicate a change in childrearing characterized by a transition from strict, patriarchal discipline of otherwise unruly children to the supervision and counselling of pliant children (Reinier 1996). The idea of a protected or sheltered childhood gained popularity in the late nineteenth century. Parents who were unable to protect their children were stigmatized (Macleod 1998). Child labour was gradually regulated in the nineteenth century and the establishment of compulsory schooling meant that school became a general feature of childhood experience by the end of the century. From the mid nineteenth century, children were being cherished by the urban middle classes for their sentimental value, within a romantic discourse of idealizing childhood (Zelizer 1985). A particular middle-class notion of childhood and family life was approved by the state as the model for working-class communities to emulate. Infant mortality was to be reduced by educating mothers in matters of hygiene and duties of care. Children's health became a state matter in response to anxieties about under-nourished children.

From the mid nineteenth century, childhood was perceived as a distinct life-cycle phase in need of intervention by charitable organizations or the state. This intervention involved an extended state surveillance of the children of poor families. The dominant approach, supported by reformers and by public opinion, was to separate children from parents in poor families. It was assumed that without their impoverished and unruly parents, children could be saved and transformed into citizens (Murdoch 2006). The strategy of nineteenth-century reformers, who identified themselves as 'child-savers', was to rescue children from their morally depraved families (Wells 2009). This view has underpinned debates about childhood in the UK and USA right up to the present day. The assumption remains that unruly children result from bad parenting rather than a combination of restricted access to material and educational resources (i.e. good housing, food, education and employment). Adequate parenting requires these basic resources. The state took on the role of 'good parent', with social problems dealt with through scientific diagnosis (Mears et al. 2007).

Children's agency

Socialization theories and sociological studies that dominated the study of children in the mid twentieth century tended to view childhood as a life phase determined not by the child's actions but by social institutions, the family or school. These approaches were critiqued by the new paradigm of childhood studies which became established by the 1990s (see James and Prout 1997). Childhood studies view childhood as a life phase shaped by children's own agency (James et al. 1998:25). The new focus on children's 'agency' has underlined the need to understand children as *social actors* who shape their own circumstances as well as being shaped by wider institutions of family and school (Qvortrup et al. 1994; Jenks 1996; Corsaro 1997; James et al. 1998; Mayall 2002; Prout 2002).

However, this new discourse of children's agency and autonomy in childhood studies has been criticized for playing down differences between children and adults. The problems surrounding the notion of children's agency are exemplified by the discourse of children's rights. Today, children are perceived to have enhanced rights, first in the form of a right to a childhood and then as a right to be treated more like adults, with access to certain privileges associated with the adult world. In addition to the United Nations Convention on the Rights of the Child, lawyers and political theorists have been concerned about attitudes of paternalism towards children and the failure by adult professionals, communities and families to acknowledge children's ability to participate as citizens autonomously (e.g. Roche 1999; Feinberg 2004). In this respect, then, the idea of *children's autonomy and rights* has important implications for parenting in contemporary families. The instatement of children's agency raises questions about how far to protect children and how far to offer them the freedom to develop their independence. Legislation passed by governments in many countries to protect children against internet child pornographers and child sex abusers does not transmit a consistent image of the rational, independent, self-directed child. In some situations, children are viewed as competent and capable of independent decision-making without parental interference, such as regarding medical treatment. In other situations, children are viewed as innocent, at risk and in need of protection against sexual and physical abuse and commercial exploitation.

The emphasis on children's agency is of particular significance for family relations and raises questions about parenting. Beck and Giddens argue, in the individualization thesis, that the status of the child is changing within new kinds of intimate relationships and new versions of family (see chapter 2). Beck (1992:18) highlights the privileged status of the child in the context of individualization and new kinds of intimacy. During late modernity, childhood is construed as 'sacred', or set apart. Contemporary ideas of childhood perceive children as special people with unique needs who need separate forms of treatment, as well as protection from the dangers and 'corrupting influences' of the adult world (see Ariès 1962; Elias 1998; James et al. 1998). From the 1970s, making friends with children as a form of 'disclosing intimacy' became a feature of the child-centred family household (Jamieson 1998). Children now occupy a central place in emotional life in the home (Jamieson 1987, 1998; Beck and Beck-Gernsheim, 1995). The child has become a sign of commitment and stability that takes precedence over the transient status of adult relationships.

Sociological research on children's family lives has foregrounded children's roles in the relational frameworks of families and confirmed their importance in shaping families (Brannen and O'Brien 1996; O'Brien et al. 1996; Dunn and Deater-Deckard 2001; Mayall 2002). Studies have also examined children's intra-family life, relationships with siblings and their friendship networks ((Edwards et al. 2005; Hey 1997; Frosh et al. 2002). Contemporary childrearing routines are set against the notion of childhood agency on the one hand, and a notion of a cherished and protected childhood on the other. This can lead to confusion for both parents and children. Since the 1970s, there has been increasing stress on children's autonomy and a corresponding decline in the value of child obedience. Over the same period, a change in professional orientation has emphasized the individualization of childhood. This entails a shift in emphasis from the aim of fitting children into society to that of providing for children in such a way as to enhance their personal development. A study of childrearing manuals in the United States across the twentieth century confirms this trend (Wrigley 1989). Professional advice from child experts shifted from an obsession with routines and processes, such as nutrition and toilet-training, to a greater stress on the need for a child's cognitive development. A range of survey data over the twentieth century indicates the corresponding changes in parenting values (Hofferth and Owens 2001). For example, fatherhood is no longer defined by its disciplining role. Today, fatherhood entails parental bonding with children through leisure. The perception that children have a right to a childhood and to have access to certain adult privileges is associated with an important change in the balance of power in families. Respect for one's elders is said to have been eroded and

apparently corresponds to the rise of youth culture, leadi..
sions in parenting. Parents are much more reluctant to use p..,
force to discipline children, especially in countries where this custo..
is now banned. It is banned in thirty countries across the world but,
notably, remains lawful in western Anglophone nations: the USA,
UK, Canada and Australia.[2]

Today's anxieties about childhood may reflect wider adult concerns
about personal identity and family stability during changing times
(Jenks 1996; Kehily 2010). Giddens argues that, like couples, parent–
child relations are being reconfigured according to the ideal of the
'pure relationship'. A transformation of intimacy and more democratic
relationships mean that children are gaining the right to 'determine
and regulate the conditions of their association' (Giddens 1992:185).
Under conditions where children are involved in decision-making,
parents now have to be answerable to them and offer them respect in
order to be respected. However, Lynn Jamieson (1998:488) reminds
us that the democratic ethic proposed by Giddens is undermined by
gendered and generational power relations in family interactions.
With mothers usually more engaged than fathers in parenting on a
daily basis, parenting is not gender-neutral. Despite mothers' efforts
to engage in mutually intimate relationships with children, mothers
and children often experience tensions over communication, disclo-
sures, surveillance and privacy (Jamieson 1999; Gillies et al. 2001). As
examples below demonstrate, these tensions often take place in the
context of the purchase of toys, use of new media in the home, wider
processes of commercialization and the privatization of home life.

Children and divorced families

Concerns about the effects of divorce on children have propelled
much of the anxiety surrounding the upbringing of children. The
number of children who experience parental divorce has inevitably
risen alongside the rise in divorce since the 1970s. For example,
over half of divorces involve couples with children under the age of
sixteen, in England and Wales. As the previous chapter shows, there
has been a particular focus on the emotional damage that parental
separation can cause children and the negative outcomes associated
with the absence of a male role model. Most research on these issues
comes from North America (see, for example, Hines 1997; Richards
1999). However, many studies tend to emphasize the impact of

parental separation on children in terms of their emotional response to parental conflict and loss, and to see this as fixed rather than as something influenced by social and economic factors. As Allan and Crow (2001:131) point out, age, gender and class are likely to mediate those experiences. Moreover, post-divorce outcomes are affected by the legal, financial and social criteria that regulate divorce in different societies.

Children's responses are influenced not only by the ending of their parents' union, but also by the behaviour of the parents towards one another both during and after the divorce. Children can find their parents' separation very distressing, and the period after the separation is one in which they often experience negative emotions and may blame themselves for the marital breakdown (Richards 1999). Parental separation is usually followed by other major changes. Many households have less income available after the separation and many face poverty (Everett 1991; Maclean 1991; Burghes 1994). The material hardships associated with separation are linked to problems in health and education (Alcock 1997; Walker and Walker 1997). Most research on the prediction of the socio-economic outcomes of divorce on children assesses the family background by using the father's characteristics (Shavit and Blossfeld 1993). However, studies in the Netherlands and Sweden found that the effects of divorce on the educational success of children appeared to depend on the pre-divorce financial and educational resources of both parents (Fischer 2007; Jonsson and Gähler 1997). Children who have fathers with a high level of these resources tend to experience greater losses *after* divorce. However, mothers with high levels of financial and educational resources tend to compensate for these losses (Fischer 2007). These indications suggest that mothers' resources should be taken into account in stratification research, given the high divorce rates across all western societies (Rowlingson and McKay 2005; Fischer 2007).

Many families move house after divorce to be nearer to other relatives or for financial reasons, which can be unsettling for the children involved. Alternatively, the parent who has left the family home, usually the father, may move far away, resulting in less contact or loss of contact with that parent (see chapter 3). This reduction in parental contact can also lead to less contact with that parent's relatives (Simpson 1998).These kinds of major changes can lead to disruptions in the lives of children at the very time when they need stability. The long-term effects of divorce on children are not easy to measure.

Initial thinking, drawn from social learning theory, about the differing effect of divorce on boys and girls was that divorce affected boys more adversely because they need a male role model in order to develop a stable masculine self-image and appropriate sex-typed behaviour (Amato and Keith 1991). It was assumed that boys are less likely to obey mothers, leading to problems of obedience. The reverse was seen to be the case for girls, since divorced mothers are more likely to be in the labour market and daughters of working mothers have higher career aspirations (Kalmijn 1994:262). More recent findings on gender differences continue to be mixed. Some studies found stronger effects for boys but others found no differences or found stronger effects for girls (Fischer 2007). Longitudinal studies suggest that divorcees are more likely to have experienced a parental divorce in childhood (Amato and DeBoer 2001). However, we have little evidence about how other factors in people's lives affect marriage and other kinds of unions. More research needs to be conducted on the effects of divorce on children to gain a clearer picture of the issues.

Children appear to deal with their parent's separation and divorce more effectively if they have positive and stable relationships with their parents (Richards 1999; Allan and Crow 2001). The tensions surrounding post-divorce parenting often concern disagreements about the organization of co-parenting after divorce (see chapter 3). Governments insist that parenting must continue after divorce. For example, the 1989 Children's Act in the UK acknowledges that divorce is the termination of marriage but not of parenting. However, Smart and Neale (1999) point out that active joint parenting, in the sense of involvement in various aspects of a child's life, entails behaviour which upholds 'family' and 'marriage', not just parenting. It involves intense levels of consultation and collaboration that depend on couples maintaining strong relations with one another. These relations are likely to be particularly difficult to maintain after divorce, especially if the divorce has been acrimonious and former spouses continue to harbour resentment. The couple may wish to distance themselves from one another while the children need them to co-parent and to continue to be tied together.

Childhood, consumption and class

Children's wish to belong and fit in with their peer group can be intense. Ethnographic work on children, inequality and consumption in the USA indicates that the desire to belong is often transformed into children's *need* to have toys, clothes and gaming systems (Chin 2001; Lareau 2003; Williams 2006; Pugh 2009). Through this desire, children place pressure on parents to spend on behalf of children. This mode of consumption has recently exploded in the USA. Key research in the USA by Allison Pugh (2009) explains the way children gain and confer dignity in order to win the right to fit in. Consumer items are central symbols for what she calls 'economies of dignity' that establish social belonging. According to Pugh, children's fear of being different from others and of either being ignored or becoming possible targets of scorn among their peers is something that concerns the parents as well as children in both affluent and low-income families. Despite very different buying practices among parents, children at both ends of the class spectrum often have similar consumer objects purchased for them. Affluent parents practise a form of 'symbolic deprivation' to express moral restraint and convey their worth as 'good' parents. Yet low-income parents apply a contrasting practice of 'symbolic indulgence' to ensure their children receive goods that have the most symbolic value (Pugh 2009:9–10).

Consumption now saturates children's relationships. Parents complain about the quantity of items that children say they need, but they also lament over the extent to which generational relations are mediated through the market. Indeed, a new category of childhood has been invented through marketing and popular culture. Pre-adolescent children are referred to as 'tweens' (Sargeant 2010) to indicate particular pre-teenage interests and target markets in toys, comics, TV programmes and video games. These trends are global. For example, research in Germany also shows how the movement from one age group to the next is handled and exhibited by children through their choice of clothes in highly individualized and unequal societies (König 2008). When they move beyond childhood, German young people enter into a finely interconnected web of rules that comprise the presentation of status distinctions and an individual self. These patterns are reflected across western countries.

The problematic roles of consumption and play in children's lives, and the way parents manage these roles, is highlighted in the UK by findings from an independently commissioned survey by the charity the Children's Society: the Good Childhood Inquiry (Layard and Dunn 2009). Corresponding with American ethnographic research on children's consumption patterns, the British survey found that having friends and spending time with them is seen as a major aspect of a good childhood by both children and parents. Yet 43 per cent of adults said that children should not be allowed out with friends until the age of fourteen. Children's desire to experience freedom appears to be impeded by parents' anxieties about giving them free movement outside the home without parental supervision. With regard to consumerism and material culture, 9 out of 10 of the 1255 adults surveyed believed that today's children are more materialistic than in previous generations. Again, this concurs with the American findings. Parents express concern at the central role that consumption plays in the formation of children's identities. Parents believe that advertising targeted at children places pressure on parents to spend more than they can afford (Layard and Dunn 2009). These kinds of studies demonstrate that consumption is a central facet of children's lives. Children and childhoods are inescapably embedded in market relations and this influences the very core of family relationships.

In addition to social class distinctions in consumption that distinguish children's social standing, parents' differing childrearing practices play a formative role in stratifying the nature, experience and quality of a child's education (Ball et al. 1996; Crozier 1996; Vincent 1996; Reay 1998). Class-related differences were identified by Annette Lareau (2002) in the 'cultural logics of childrearing', confirming that social class influences patterns of family life. Middle-class parenting entails a 'concerted cultivation' of children. Middle-class parents 'enrol their children in numerous age-specific, organized activities that dominate family life and create enormous labour, particularly for mothers. The parents view these activities as transmitting life skills to children' (Lareau 2002:748). By contrast, the childrearing strategies of the working-class and poor parents tend to emphasize the accomplishment of 'natural growth'. Working-class parents do not focus on developing their children's special talents, believing that as long as they provide love, food and safety, their children will grow and thrive.

This distinction between *concerted cultivation* and *natural growth* is also supported by Carol Vincent and Stephen Ball (2006, 2007) who studied middle-class and working-class parents' use and choice of childcare. They refer to the construction of the 'renaissance child' through the provision of 'enrichment' activities, involving extra-curricular sports and creative classes in which families enrol their children, mostly those less than five years old. They found that working-class parents are less likely to afford these activities and classes and are less likely to see their children as a project for development. They are more likely to perceive their children's characteristics, skills and talent as less flexible and more static. The investment of time and money by middle-class parents is a major way of enhancing middle-class privilege, indicating the extent that middle-class parents go to in creating strategies for class reproduction (Griffith and Smith 2005). This middle-class investment in a child's future is referred to as *cultural capital* (Bourdieu 1983) and is gender-specific as well as class-specific. Cultural capital is a resource or set of values and knowledges that confers advantage. It refers to the educational, intellectual and cultural assets imparted by the family to their child to foster upward social mobility. Mothers take the responsibility for researching, arranging and monitoring the care and education of the children, and their attendance at activities (Vincent and Ball 2007), and for developing the 'learning readiness' of pre-school children (Griffith and Smith 2005). The purchase of expertise through recreational activities, tutoring or parenting classes is the most obvious way in which cultural capital is linked to economic capital (Bourdieu 2004:19). In these ways, culture is used by parents as a *resource* to generate the 'middle-class self' in the child.

The concerted cultivation used by middle-class parents to provide their children with cultural capital lies at the very heart of liberal individualism. The *renaissance child* is equipped with the skills to make choices and realize their inherent capabilities or potential and become a self-developing subject (Skeggs 2004; Vincent and Ball 2007). The renaissance child develops intellectual, creative and sporting skills and experiences derived from a large number of activities – such as music, drama or French classes – which are undertaken around the ages of three to five with diverse developmental and investment purposes. The aim is to prepare the child for future success at school and therefore in their eventual career. Although not exclusively middle-class, the bounded settings of these life-skill classes are part of a 'social cocooning' of children which often sets limits on social mixing. Even older children tend to be escorted or driven to these enrichment activities by their parents. Vincent and Ball (2007) conclude that these activities are a response to the anxiety and sense of responsibility experienced by middle-class parents as they attempt to 'make up' a middle-class child in a social context in which the reproduction of privilege may appear uncertain.

These views concur with the work of Margaret Nelson (2010) who has identified a new kind of 'parenting out of control'. Children of the elite suffer out-of-control parents, whom she refers to as 'helicopter parents'. In her analysis of the aspirations American parents have for their children, and the strategies they use to realize them, Nelson identifies major class differences in parenting styles. She contrasts 'parenting out of control' with 'parenting with limits' to address the apparent failure by parents in their attempts to set realistic boundaries in raising their children. Nelson identifies the stereotypes and media exaggerations about today's prosperous, well-educated American parents. Parents who prepare their children for competition and new challenges of life feel they must remain attentive and alert, hover, interfere and guide the child (Nelson 2010). These 'helicopter' elite and middle-class parents are perceived to be stifling their children's development and creating infantilized, spoiled, immature adults who become ill-equipped to cope with the real world.

Thus, 'parenting out of control' indicates excessive parental influence among 'elite', well-resourced, families. This parenting style involves the enrolment of children in a wide range of extracurricular activities and assessment of all academic achievement. Echoing the 'concerted cultivation' mentioned above, Nelson records the way elite American parents plan schedules designed to help secure the child a competitive place in the world, affecting every area of the child's life. This depth of parental influence involves the building of relationships with children based on intimacy, on being available, on staying connected, on intense supervision and on friendship. It also involves shielding the middle-class child from the external constraints generally imposed on children 'Parenting out of control' relies, then, on the availability of enormous amounts of time and money to support an elite style of care.

The children of the elite gain access to a wide range of resources such as private college coaches, tutoring for exams, and excellent schools. New technologies such as cell phones, social networking sites and even GPS devices provide parents with more opportunities to communicate with, supervise and spy on their children, yet often contribute to 'parenting out of control'. The effect is persistent surveillance of a highly personalized, negotiated and continuous nature. By contrast, 'parenting with limits' refers to a parenting style with less intense relationships. It allows children more flexibility to explore and develop their own identities. It involves clearer restrictions on behaviour, and more clearly defined parameters on the time and energy devoted to parenting. Nelson found that lower-income students had to earn significant amounts of money to ease the economic burden on their parents of the costs of having a child in college. Occasionally, they were even sending money to their parents, indicating that, for them, support was reciprocal.

Children, new media and the home

Another area of rising tension between parents and children is children's use of new media in the home. The introduction of a wide range of media gadgets into the home has prompted renegotiations of household relationships between children and parents. These renegotiations have been complicated by the uncertainties and disagreements which surround the rights and responsibilities of children. The growth in home-based media use by children has coincided with the rise of youth-centred media and a screen-rich 'bedroom culture' (Bovill and Livingstone 2001; Lincoln 2004; Livingstone 2009). Today, adolescents spend significant amounts of their leisure time in the privacy of bedrooms, rather than in communal family spaces, through the solitary use of new media (Bovill and Livingstone 2001; Livingstone 2002). In this private space, children are more likely to be in communication with a virtual, outside world beyond the home, through the internet, than with adult members of their own household. Parents often joke that they have to text their children to gain their attention at mealtimes. The solitary use of media gadgets by children and teenagers seems to indicate an individualization of media use in the home and a fragmentation of domestic leisure between young people and adults (Flichy 1995; Mackay 1997; Livingstone 2002). New patterns of family associations are being identified, described as 'living together but separately' (Flichy 1995; van Rompaey and Roe 2001). Emergent types of interaction and regulation in households are being created by parents who feel obliged to restrict the extent to which their children use phones, computers, the internet, video games, etc. (Silverstone and Haddon 1996; Haddon 2004).

The increase in new media items in children's bedrooms at younger and younger ages has fuelled public anxieties about children and media use (Critcher 2008; Livingstone 2009). In the Good Childhood Enquiry, most parents agreed that children's television and computer time should be restricted, and that violent video games make children more violent (Layard and Dunn 2009). Media panics persist about socially disengaged young people replacing human contact with virtual contact. The idea of a risk-averse culture is supported by some negative research findings. The tendency for adolescents to be separated from adult life can be accelerated by new media use (Drotner et al. 2008; Subrahmanyam and Greenfield 2008). On the one hand, extensive use of information communication technologies (ICTs) by young people has been associated with poor health, the decline of face-to-face communication, social isolation, low self-esteem and social incompetence (Strasbourg and Wilson 2002; Gentile et al. 2004; Vandebosch and Van Cleemput 2009). On the other hand, more positive research findings suggest greater teen autonomy, greater teen choice, and enhancement of peer group relations (Buckingham 2007; Heim et al. 2007; Cheong 2008; Livingstone 2009; Patchin and Hinduja 2010). Nevertheless, tensions between parents and children over young people's uses of new media are accelerating. Parental control is declining as the technology becomes more complicated and unfamiliar (Livingstone 2009). Parents are concerned about losing control over children's lives and being unable to protect them against problems such as cyberbullying and game violence.

Yet parents are frequently poorly informed about their children's activities and often fail to monitor them effectively (Subrahmanyam and Greenfield 2008; Ulicsak and Cranmer 2010). The entry of new ICTs into the home affects people's relationships with existing media technologies. Linking games consoles to the main family TV set often generates disagreements between parents and children (Haddon 2006:116). However, other evidence suggests that games consoles gravitate into the private space of children's bedrooms, with 69 per cent of 5–to 16–year-olds in the UK having games consoles, radios and DVD players in their bedrooms (ChildWise 2009). Parents feel pressured to make deals with their children about when and where they can play video and computer games, such as after completion of school homework (Silverstone 2006). Parent–child collaborative video gaming is now regarded as a major mediating strategy for parents (Nikken et al. 2007). The launch of family-centred video gaming during a climate of moral uncertainty and familial changes has tremendous appeal, especially since the new youth leisure technology market is mostly financed by parents. Family gaming such as Nintendo Wii, Microsoft Xbox and Sony Playstation claims to offer parents opportunities for both family bonding and control of children's use of new media (Chambers 2011).

Parents highlight benefits from playing video games together as a family when the games selected emphasize parental monitoring or guidance roles and skills teaching. However, parent–child bonding through gaming is largely with primary-school-aged children. Adolescents continue to be mainly solitary players (Ulicsak et al. 2009). Young people in general continue to play alone much more than with their parents (Dromgoole 2009). Teenagers desire independence to be able to play games away from parental supervision. They often feel a strong sense of invasion of privacy if parents wander into their territory (Horst 2008). Such attitudes among young people are likely to represent a major challenge for family relationships in general. The issue of 'disengaged youth' may be a persistent problem, regardless of family-centred new media. How the family interacts around the gaming activities also appears to depend on pre-existing family relationships (Ulicsak and Cranmer 2010:17).

The privatization of childhood

In certain parts of the non-western world, the concept of 'childhood' appears to be changing through an extension of western, privatized and individualized family life. The privatization of childhood and children's growing seclusion in the home in contemporary urban China may offer an insight into the way these changes are spreading in urban contexts transnationally (Naftali 2010). The recent recognition of Chinese children's right to privacy is being promoted by public discourses and incorporated in everyday life. The state still plays a key role in the urban Chinese family life, including its 'one-child' population policy (see chapter 7). However, in the past few decades the private sphere has been identified as the main context for socializing China's children (Anagnost 2008). The escalation of market reforms from the 1990s coincides with a shift from state dependence to self-reliance among China's citizens (Woronov 2007:30; Ong and Zhang 2008:8).

During this period, popular childrearing literature increased in China. Urban parents, especially mothers, are called upon by the state to take responsibility for 'realizing the potentiality for value' in their single child (Anagnost 2008:60). However, the accent on children's right to 'individual privacy' (*geren yinsi*), materially and psychologically, has been accompanied by a growing physical seclusion of urban Chinese children in the home. Chinese concepts of privacy and childhood underwent a dramatic change in the twentieth century. Most urban Chinese children did not have access to their own room until recently. The notion of 'private' gradually took on positive connotations and was linked with changing ideas about the individual and the nuclear family. In order to foster a modern, self-assured and patriotic citizenry, Chinese reformers in the late twentieth century reflected western ideas of childhood agency, advancing the notion that children and youth form a distinct social group. Its distinctiveness can be articulated through separate existence and private wishes in their relation to parents and the extended family (Farquhar 1999; Jones 2002). A growing number of urban Chinese families are buying their own homes as a consequence of the reduction in family size resulting from the 'one-child' policy, the privatization of the housing market, growing family incomes and rising consumption (Naftali 2010). However, this trend towards the privatization of childhood has coincided with a significant restriction of children's mobility. Interestingly, the similarity in trends in childhoods between urban China and western societies, with childhood set apart as unique and special, reveals key ambiguities and problems about the contradictions between ideas of childhood agency and freedom on the one hand, and increasing privatization and confinement of childhood on the other. This management of childhood is generated, then, by both state and commercial interests.

Although childhood is regarded as one of the most regulated phases of personal life, Nicolas Rose (1999) explains that in Europe and North America the surveillance of childhood has shifted from the state to families. The contemporary family now conducts a form of self-regulation away from the intrusion of state and market relations in what Rose refers to as a 'strategy of family privacy'. The trend of childhood privatization in urban China suggests that the Chinese family is also embracing this western strategy of self-regulation, away from state scrutiny. The principle of family privacy in the West, which is spreading to other urban centres, is proof of past state successes in forging the kind of family that would, of its own accord, take responsibility for the duties of socialization by *internalizing* the morals and values associated with those duties as its own aspirations (Rose 1999:213). Thus, the raft of professionals that once monitored the family in a coercive way – such as the police, social workers and probation officers – no longer need to. Instead, families are addressed by health advisors, counsellors, teachers and other experts through magazines, books, TV and radio, 'and through the unceasing reflexive gaze of our own psychologically educated self-scrutiny' (Rose 1999:213). Family self-surveillance is prompted by the ambition to be a 'good family', and a central feature of this ambition is the 'correct' family regulation of childhood through customs and practices that show both respect for and control of children.

Conclusions

This chapter has shown that the notion of children's self-determination and rights has dramatic implications for the 'new parenting' of the late modern era. Certain features of these changes seem to be contradictory. On the one hand, there is a new period of 'extended youth' in which children are expected to be more autonomous and self-directed, with an apparent loosening of parental supervision in and out of the home (Livingstone 2009). On the other hand, young people stay at home and remain financially dependent on their parents for longer periods than in the past. This can lead to tensions in parenting and in children's identities due to the differing expectations about the amount of guidance and disciplining entailed in the upbringing of children. Transformations in family arrangements characterized by rising divorce rates and post-divorce and 'new' families have generated public anxieties about a crisis of commitment to children and can lead to tensions in parent–child relationships. Children are no longer treated as the passive recipients of parental care and socialization. They are now acknowledged as moral and social practitioners of family life in their own right.

Prompted by the belief that children should have a personal space in the private family household, a noticeable trend towards the *privatization* of childhood coincides with a restriction on children's mobility. The similarities in models of childhood between urban China and western societies, where childhood is treated as distinctive and exceptional, are striking. They signify uncertainties about the contemporary status of childhood, expressed through a tension between notions of childhood agency and childhood management and new kinds of family life.

The move towards child-centred family households, in which children have a central role in emotional life, coincides with anxieties about children's use of media in the home. The home has become a youth-centred, media-rich space for children in affluent western nations. However, debates about children's use of ITCs in the home epitomize the tensions associated with concepts of childhood agency and the need for parental protection. A new kind of childhood has emerged, one securely embedded in the family home yet potentially in communication with a worldwide network of friends. Outside the home, children's consumption and use of specific commodities have become an essential aspect of a child's integration into a peer group and progression through the stages of the life-cycle. Progression through the phases of childhood, for example from childhood to adolescence, is displayed by the use of certain brands, styles of clothing and personalized mobile media gadgets such as mobile phones.

As we have seen, the expediency of contemporary childrearing practices which are set against the romantic ideal and the rights discourse can cause concern for parents and children, particularly during periods of dramatic disruption such as divorce. The idea of childhood as innocent and vulnerable is highlighted by research on the effects of divorce on children. However, more research is needed to understand how children manage life in post-divorce and blended families, particularly when they are transferred between two or more 'homes' in order to retain contact with estranged parents. The rights framework of thinking promoted by the new sociology of childhood has coincided with an important change in the balance of power in families, between parents and children. Yet the challenges of negotiating disruptions in family life have not been centrally addressed by this new paradigm, despite the fact that children become more visible after divorce.

5 Families and Ageing Societies

The realization that western nations are now 'ageing societies' has led to heated debates about the role of families and the state in caring for older people. These are problems related to the financial costs of an ageing society. Changes in family obligations over the life course have been driven not only by increases in life expectancy and the rise in the number and age of elderly people but also by an extension of the age of reproduction, longer periods of life after parenting and rising divorce rates. There are several key factors affecting families in relation to ageing. First, in western nations, the widening geographical distance between natal and marital homes triggered by geographical mobility and migration is influencing the kind of childcare support *given* by grandparents and the form of care being *received* by the elderly. Second, the decrease in state welfare provision is affecting family duties and intergenerational relations, raising issues about the adequacy of household resources in relation to wider social welfare provision. A third issue is that older women tend to live longer than men. Many of the problems associated with ageing, reduced welfare provision and accelerated poverty in old age are affecting women more directly than men. A fourth trend is a forging of new social ties by families and older people to cope with the caring responsibilities of an ageing society in an era characterized by smaller families, weaker extended kinship ties, rising numbers of single-person households and same-sex couple relationships. Various new configurations of social support beyond the family, including friends, neighbours and extended kin, are involved in caring for elderly members of society.

This chapter explores the impact of ageing and retirement on family structures and experiences in western cultures by addressing these patterns of change. The chapter also addresses the interplay of ageing, family change and policy reform in a global context, by examining the challenges of ageing, poverty and migration for non-western societies. The examples drawn on from different regions reflect the major research on ageing and intergenerational relations in the context of policy studies, gerontology and development studies.

Changing dynamics of ageing and family life in western societies

'Population ageing' is a term used to describe the situation in societies where older people, usually identified as those aged over sixty or sixty-five, comprise a higher proportion of the total population than do the young and middle-aged. As a widespread phenomenon, population ageing is generating new challenges and leading to new patterns of family reciprocity in many societies. However, the older population is not a uniform group. Since women, on average, live longer than men they comprise the majority of older people, in a process known as the 'feminization of later life'. This trend reflects a steep decline in fertility and mortality rates. In developed nations, sociological studies have extended attention from male retirement as a defining characteristic of the 'problem of old age', to include the demographic feminization of the aged population. This development has led to an increase in studies of the circumstances and experiences of older women (Russell 2007).

The problems of population ageing coincide directly with the shrinkage in welfare provision by states in western nations. Governments expect families, however defined, to take increasing responsibility for the caring of elderly relatives at a time when families themselves are undergoing rapid change and facing economic hardships prompted by a world recession. The mid-twentieth-century emergence of the European social security systems was part of an expansion of social rights that embraced citizens' welfare in these comparatively wealthy nations. Historically, European citizenship conceived of people as rights-bearing, self-directed individuals The contractual relations between the state and individuals entailed welfare provision for those in need, from cradle to grave. Thus, welfare provision became the duty of the state towards the individual, leading to the establishment of a mainly public-sectored welfare system.

Public pension schemes in western nations are in a state of crisis since they cannot be sustained without economic growth and productivity to meet the needs of the population ageing process (Hock

Guan 2008). European countries have been forced to reconsider their policies and programmes by increasing the age of retirement. Since 2006, tens of thousands of people across Western Europe have been protesting against these pension reforms. This is because older workers continue to be at risk of being fired because of their age. Many middle-aged workers therefore perceive themselves to be at risk of poverty because they are regarded as too old to work and yet too young to receive state pension (Greenberg and Muehlebach 2007).

Within debates about the role and extent of social welfare support to be given to families in caring for an ageing population, certain researchers point to a recent 're-medicalization' of old age in western societies (Means 2007). This perspective tends to present a 'welfare model' of older families to highlight questions about who is responsible for caring for the elderly and older families. The welfare perspective has tended to ignore the differing experiences of living in families with older members, in terms of roles and relationships. Pat Chambers and colleagues (2009) argue that more attention should be paid to the complexity of experiences of older families and the diverse family practices among older people. Changing western family forms and values have generated significant diversity in experiences of ageing. Despite major transformations in family life, older people are often still depicted as having limited options and little control over their lives. While poverty and ill health can seriously restrict the choices of older people, many are no more dependent than younger people. They are just as likely to be engaged in a variety of interdependent relationships that include friends and family members. Within the constraints of their material circumstances, they exercise agency over their lifestyle choices (Chambers et al. 2009).

Older people and patterns of family support

By studying long-term trends in family ties and friendships in America since the 1970s, Claude Fischer (2011) found that Americans have fewer relatives today than in previous decades and that formal family gatherings have declined over the years. To some extent, this trend is as a result of later marriages, more single-parent families, and the rise in the number of employed women. However, in terms of the effects on type and quality of support for older people, changes in living arrangements and the proximity of family households have been major factors. In 1900 in the United States, more than 60 per cent of those aged sixty-five and above lived with one or more of their children. The elderly shared their resources with their offspring. Living alone in old age continued to be exceptional in the mid twentieth century, whereas today's older people are now much more likely to live on their own or with a spouse rather than in a household with their adult children. The western trend towards small, nuclear, independent households from the early 1960s involved an increase in the number of people living alone and a decline in those living with members of kin other than their spouse. Improved personal financial resources and broader housing options encouraged the rise of separate residences. By the mid-1970s, the proportion of older Americans who lived with their children dropped to just 14 per cent (Haber and Gratton 1994). These trends were echoed in the UK. By the 1990s, only 5 per cent of older people in the UK lived with an adult child, compared to 40 per cent at start of the 1950s (Wall 1998). In today's Britain, the most recent census data indicated that 37 per cent of older people lived alone (Office for National Statistics 2001).

Although more than a third of older people live alone today in western societies, there are significant gender and age variations. Elderly men are much more likely than elderly women to live with their spouses, since they tend to die at a younger age than women. Older women are likely to outlive their spouses and live alone after the death of their husband. Of women aged seventy-five and over, 60 per cent now live alone compared with 29 per cent of men of the same age (Thompson 1994). However, there are significant ethnic variations in household living arrangements. Multi-generational households are now uncommon except among certain ethnic minority groups, such as South Asians and Chinese. Among these and other ethnic groups, a higher proportion of older people tend to live in complex households, with more than one generation. For example, in the UK, 42 per cent of South Asian men aged eighty-five and over lived in a complex household, compared with 12 per cent of white men in the 2001 Census. Among women, the equivalent figures were 68 per cent of South Asian women aged eighty-five living with relatives, compared to 19 per cent of white women (Soule et al. 2005).

Residential proximity between older people and their kin has also altered considerably since the 1950s. The British post-war studies confirmed that it was common for older people to have at least one relative living within a mile of their home. Today, close relationships are more geographically dispersed. A British survey of 2007 found that 44 per cent of respondents over the age of seventy had no close relative living nearby (Cabinet Office 2008). The question is whether the greater distances between kin have substantially changed the family life of older people. High levels of geographical mobility mean that elderly relatives live farther away from their adult children than fifty years ago, so families have to travel significant distances to maintain face-to-face contact. However, older people tend to remain part of a significant kinship network made up of children, grandchildren and siblings as well as spouses or partners (Phillipson et al. 2001). Research indicates that levels of interaction between older people and their families continue to be extensive. In Britain, a survey in 2004 reported that three-quarters of older people, 77 per cent, saw relatives at least weekly, with just around 1 in 10 seeing relatives less than once a year (Victor et al. 2004). British South Asian families tend to care for the elderly within the same home as extended kinship networks (Russell 2007). In the United States, elderly parents with health problems tend to move closer to their children to benefit from their support (Longino et al. 1991; Serow and Sly 1991). Despite greater distances between older and younger family members, the family remains a crucial source of support to older people when there are particular needs such as household tasks, help when ill, and talking over emotional problems.

Many families also maintain contact with close relatives over long distances through communication technologies such as email and skyping. Evidence suggests that the types of relationships that people build up are more varied nowadays, with family formations changing over the life course. Many older people rely on friendship networks for practical and emotional support, as well as kin (Adams and Blieszner 1989; Phillipson et al. 2001). This is more common among those who are single, widowed or childless, and also among middle-class and professional groups. It is also expected to increase as a characteristic of future cohorts. Networks of choice, consisting of ties of friendship as well as relationships of kin, are on the increase (Spencer and Pahl 2006; see chapter 9). Fischer (2010) draws the conclusion that the overall quantity of today's personal relationships and the quality of those relationships have not necessarily diminished.

With regard to the influence of state welfare on intergenerational family ties and the commitment to provide financial support and care, it was feared that tensions would arise between 'welfare generations' in European countries in the 1980s and 1990s (Kohli et al. 2000). However, the generations appear to be maintaining their commitment to each other. Associations between parents and adult children involve a significant amount of reciprocal support of a financial, instrumental and social kind (Arber and Attias-Donfut 1999; Bonvalet and Ogg 2007; and Hoff and Tesch-Romer 2007). A study of cross-national variations in family relationships in European countries and Israel examined variations in attitudes to care for older people between England, Germany, Spain, Israel and Norway (Lowenstein and Daatland 2006). The evidence suggests that public welfare support has tended to *strengthen* rather than lessen family solidarity. Support was also regularly provided by older relatives to younger family members. Attitudes about the degree of care that adult children should provide for ageing parents tended to vary along north–south lines. Support was highest in Spain and Israel and rather lower in Norway, England and Germany (Lowenstein and Daatland 2006). The geographical proximity of adult children and their parents showed a similar north–south divide, greatest in Spain and Israel and least in Norway. In Spain and Israel, most respondents agreed that adult children should live near their parents, whereas the English and, particularly, the Norwegians emphasized living independently (Daatland and Herlofson 2003).

While there has been extensive research on family care within the majority white population of the UK, there is less understanding of the family care provision for its growing older ethnic population. However, research is now uncovering evidence that older members of minority ethnic groups, such as those who experienced migration, are more susceptible to poverty and social exclusion in old age. For example, migrants from the Caribbean and Indian subcontinent to the UK in the 1950s, who are now reaching old age, are often in difficult financial and personal circumstances. Minority ethnic groups such as Pakistanis and Bangladeshis are more likely to have been unemployed before retirement than their white counterparts. They are more likely to have suffered from ill health and to be experiencing poverty in their older years (Nazroo et al. 2004). High levels of poverty were found among older people from certain minority ethnic groups who lived in inner-city areas, particularly among Somalis (77 per cent of whom were in poverty) and Pakistanis (67 per cent) (Scharf et al. 2002). Such circumstances are likely to worsen, given the social pressures associated with growing levels of unemployment and the low level of income from supplementary pensions (Chambers et al.

2009; Phillipson 2009). Reduced welfare provision in western nations is likely to generate new vulnerabilities associated with poverty and poor housing for older people, notably women and those from ethnic minorities.

Much research on grandparenting since the early 1990s, particularly in the USA, indicates a growing recognition of the considerable amount of grandparenting that families benefit from (Minkler 1999; Goodman and Silverstein 2001). It demonstrates clearly that older people are not simply a liability to younger family members and the state. Across the world, grandparents supply vital childcare, allowing mothers to enter paid work. The extent of grandparental childcare provision and childrearing advice also undermines claims of family decline. Women are much more involved in grandparenting than men due to the greater responsibilities they normally take on for domestic organization and family relationships. Echoing the findings of earlier, mid-twentieth-century studies of traditional working-class communities, intergenerational female kinship networks remain essential forms of domestic and familial organization (Young and Willmott 1957, 1987; Rosser and Harris 1965, 1983; Bell 1968; Leonard 1980). Across societies, grandparents' interest in their grandchildren is validated through cultural norms of intergenerational 'blood' connection with expectations of grandparental wisdom, emotional attachment and involvement (Chambers et al. 2009). Nonetheless, this role is changing. In terms of demographic circumstances, people become grandparents at younger ages, in their fifties. However, with the latest western trend of marriage and/or having children later in life, this pattern is altering (Dench and Ogg 2002). In late modernity, not only is the provision of practical help often hampered by geographical distance – many grandparents are still in full-time employment and likely to have active social lives.

Changes in household arrangements since the early 1970s, exemplified by rising divorce rates, cohabitation, lone parenthood and remarriage, have led to more diverse circumstances in the roles of grandparents. As the quality of the relationship between the grandparent and grandchild depends on the quality of the relationship with the child's parents, parental separation or divorce can place a strain on grandparent–grandchild contact (Mueller and Elder 2003; Ferguson et al. 2004). When a non-resident parent, usually the father, loses touch with his children through divorce or separation, the grandparents usually become estranged too. Maternal grandparents tend to be more involved by providing practical, financial, emotional support for their daughter and grandchildren in the period following separation or divorce (Ferguson et al. 2004).

Gender differences among older people

Issues of gender, salient to the sociology of ageing, have undergone a notable transformation in the last fifty years. The loss of the role of paid work for older people was regarded as a major crisis of identity in the mid twentieth century. Since work was a role central to men's identities, the 'problem of old age' was seen as the problem of old men, as exemplified by the work of Parsons (1942). Ageing women were assumed to experience continuity of identity through the ongoing performance of their key role of domestic reproduction and could therefore safely be ignored (Jones et al. 2010:112). By the 1970s, feminist scholars began to question the preoccupation with men's retirement as the key problem of old age, highlighting its 'masculinist bias' in gerontological research. It is now well recognized that women are significantly worse off after retirement than men. They tend to be poorer, have access to fewer resources from the state, and yet live longer. Drawing attention to the fact that women comprise the numerically larger group of older persons, feminist research has documented the many disadvantages faced by older women, particularly the greater risk of poverty, widowhood, poor health and institutionalization (e.g. Beeson 1975; Russell 1987). By the 1990s, claims that the issues associated with ageing are more frequently 'women's issues' had become commonplace (see, for example, Arber and Ginn 1991; Heycox 1997).

From an initial research focus on male retirement as the defining characteristic of the 'problem of old age', then, sociological studies now acknowledge a demographic feminization of the aged population by focusing on the circumstances and experiences of the numerically larger group of older women (Russell 2007). Since women live longer, they are more likely to need formal care services for longer periods than men. Gender differences in disability and the numerical imbalance between women and men in later life means that the provision and receipt of informal care are gendered. Older women are therefore more likely than older men to have their activities of daily living impaired by functional disabilities. Yet women are far less likely to have a spouse to provide care and enable them to remain living in the community. Married men can generally rely on their wives when care is required, with all the advantages this brings, whereas women are more likely to have to call upon adult children for help. Women are also twice as likely as men to enter residential care (Ginn and Arber 1995:10–11).

In terms of the caring needs of older people, women face distinctive problems. The disadvantages of old age and sacrifices made by women throughout their lives include low-paid, part-time work; poor superannuation; and taking time out from employment for child-rearing or caring for elderly relatives. In addition, women sacrifice promotion and career security to follow husbands' employment-led relocation (Chapman 2004). Since women are notably poorer after retirement than men, the accelerated and global decline in state welfare provision is expected to increase the burden of care for ageing relatives on younger women. Against the background of reduced public spending from the mid-1970s, older people began to be seen as a financial drain on western economies (Fennell et al. 1988:52). Financial savings were sought by reducing the most expensive, institutional forms of aged care. Transferring an increasing number and range of medical services and conditions into the family home became an explicit policy goal of western governments. Since older women were the most affected group, the vast majority of recipients of residential and community aged care services are elderly widowed women. By contrast, the costs of caring for elderly men are more likely to be borne privately through the unpaid labour of their wives who outlive them (Chapman 2004).

Same-sex relationships among older people

New forms of intimacy and new living arrangements are taking place among older lesbians and gay men. Those now reaching old age represent a generation who experienced a society in which same-sex relationships were criminalized and pathologized (Heaphy et al. 2003). Many LGBT elders may therefore be less open about their sexual orientation than younger generations. In their lifetime, there have been unprecedented changes in societal attitudes and legislation around sexual orientation, as chapter 3 describes. Research about same-sex partnerships indicates that they often do not conform to gender stereotypes associated with the traditional gendered norms in households structured by inequalities of labour, resources, status and power. As mentioned in chapter 2, non-heterosexual couples are more likely to experience relationships guided by values of egalitarianism, independence and agency when freed from the conventions of gender inequality. However, some older LGBT couples' relationships have been affected by former heterosexual relationships (Heaphy et al. 2004).

Older LGBT men and women are more likely to live alone than their heterosexual counterparts and this mode of living increases with age (Brookdale Center on Aging 1999; Cahill et al. 2000; Heaphy et al. 2003; de Vries 2007). However, estimating the size and demographic trends of the ageing LGBT population is difficult with no official UK demographic statistics on LGBT individuals of any age group. In the UK, the Department of Trade and Industry (DTI) (2003) estimates that the ageing LGBT population comprises 5–7 per cent nationally. While the individualization thesis has influenced sociological debates about the diversity of family forms, Brian Heaphy (2009) questions its applicability to older LGBT generations. Research on non-heterosexual older men and women has highlighted the value placed on sustained relationships in later life (Heaphy et al. 2004; Porche and Purvin 2008).

Although little research has been conducted on how illness and disability are managed in long-lasting non-heterosexual relationships, Heaphy and colleagues (2004) have identified the importance of a partner as a key support in the event of illness. They also found that older non-heterosexual men and women lack trust in formal services. Formal services tend to be dominated by heteronormative assumptions or predicated around beliefs about the asexuality of older people and are therefore less likely to provide appropriate and sensitive support to gay and lesbian older couples facing illness or disability. Older non-heterosexual men and women may have spent their adult lives making complex decisions and choices about whether or not and to whom they reveal their sexuality. More research is needed on how ageing shapes the experiences of providing and receiving care within non-heterosexual intimate relationships (Heaphy et al. 2004).

Sexual orientation can influence the quality of social support available to individuals towards the end of life. Research on end of life care continues to focus mainly on family relationships, with a particular emphasis on family support and care giving. Yet there is also a continuing bias in favour of families constructed by marriage or blood ties in much research (Manthorpe 2003). The ageing LGBT population in the UK is a significant minority with particular end of life care needs and concerns to address (Almack et al. 2010). The End of Life Care Strategy in England which studied the needs of the LGBT population in relation to end of life care found that sexual orientation is one of the most likely areas for inequality and discrimination to occur in end of life care (Department of Health 2008).

A study by Brotman et al. (2003) indicates that relatives have, in the past, offered little support or even shown hostility to their LGBT kin and their partners. Disclosure of one's sexual orientation may lead to estrangement from families of origin, leading LGBT individuals to depend on and prefer alternative support networks. The wider neglect, in research, of the role of friendship and informal social networks has also been noted (Young et al. 1998). A small-scale British study of how sexual orientation may impact on concerns about, and experiences of, end of life care and bereavement within same-sex relationships, by Almack, Seymour and Bellamy (2010), showed that friends as family, chosen families, were vital. These chosen families have been described as fluid but 'often strong and supportive networks of friends, lovers and even family of origin' which create a framework for mutual care for many lesbians and gay men (Weeks et al.1999b:44).

When a partner dies, disenfranchisement can occur in non-traditional relationships, such as a same-sex relationship, that are not fully recognized or where the couple has not disclosed their relationship to others. However, it is likely that future generations of LGBT elders may be more open and confident about disclosing their sexual orientation and will expect services to address their particular needs (Almack et al. 2010). A British study of same-sex commitment ceremonies that considers the significance of the recently introduced Civil Partnership Act (2005) suggests that it may encourage new forms of kinship to develop as same-sex partners are brought into the wider family, and 'in-laws' could come together to form extended families too (Shipman and Smart 2007). Non-kin ties are becoming increasingly important for older people. In her work on lesbian relationships, Gillian Dunne (1997) suggests that, while traditionally gendered heterosexual couples may be characterized as 'intimate strangers', couples in same-sex relationships can be more accurately portrayed as 'intimate friends'. Research on long-lasting non-heterosexual relationships, both lesbian and gay, has highlighted the significance of friendship principles in shaping and sustaining these ties (Johnson 1990; Heaphy et al. 1999; Budgeon 2006).

Non-kin ties are likely to dominate in later life in future among heterosexual as well as LGBT couples. However, little is known about the dynamics and experiences of friendship links across generations (Almack et al. 2010). It seems likely, though, that the increasing diversity of current marriage and partnership behaviour will correspond with more diverse personal networks in later life. Friendship is now playing a key role in the lives of older people by providing emotional support and practical forms of assistance once typically offered by family members (Adams and Blieszner 1989; Phillipson et al. 2001). The centrality of kinship that once characterized older people's lives is shifting to networks of 'choice' consisting of ties to friends, leisure associates and neighbours as well as family relationships (Chambers 2006; Spencer and Pahl 2006). This theme is revisited in chapter 9. However, as the next section indicates, in non-western parts of the world a new kind of ageing is being generated by globalization, in circumstances where interpersonal relationships are often shaped by very different kinds of values.

Globalization, old age and traditional kinship customs

Global differences in attitudes and values about 'family' and the social obligations associated with caring impact on experiences of ageing. In many non-western regions, such as East and Southeast Asian countries, individuals are regarded as *role-bearing* and *family-directed* rather than *rights-bearing* and *autonomous*. In comparison with the West, greater importance is generally placed on tangible interpersonal relationships which define the person's social status. The community, and particularly the family, are assigned central roles in this social contract (Hock Guan 2008). For example, in East and Southeast Asian countries, the family and wider kinship networks make major inputs into the care of the elderly (Hatmadji and Wiyono 2008; Mehta and Leng 2008; Natividad 2008). However, traditionally family-based systems of welfare have been compromised in many developing countries by a number of new, westernized trends, including the changing views about family roles, the rise in nuclear families and unmarried adults, a reduction in fertility rates and accelerated population mobility. In Southeast Asian countries, for example, these social shifts place tremendous pressure on governments to perform a greater future role in the care of the elderly and to take such factors into account in the development of income security schemes for old age (Hock Guan 2008).

The subject of ageing is currently generating active discussion in China. The circumstances in China, with its 'one-child' policy (see chapter 7), remind us that ageing populations are not only a concern for the more-developed countries. The lack of social security programmes and pension arrangements in China has prompted the spread of laws such as the 1997 Family Law, which seeks to make the care of elderly parents the *legal duty* of adult children. Previously, this was part of the socio-Confucian value system which traditionally lay at the heart of Chinese society. But when combined with fertility decline and rising life expectancies, the effects of the reform era in China have put a strain on traditional value systems and resulted in cases of parent-abandonment. China is just one example of a society in the so-called 'developing world' having to face up to the prospects of population ageing.

Global transformations in ageing are increasingly coinciding with changing intergenerational family dynamics, fertility, migration, gender roles and social policy (Izuhara 2010). Rising transnational migration, prompted by poverty and the search for employment, is coinciding with a fragmentation of family ties by often eroding or compromising forms of reciprocal arrangements customary in generational relations (see chapter 6). Migration is therefore raising important questions about the political economy of informal and formal care of the elderly, as well as the young (Torres 2006; Chambers et al. 2009:96; Phillipson 2010). In this section, a number of examples across the developing world are addressed to provide an idea of some of the regional variations in family approaches to ageing. For example, developing countries such as those in sub-Saharan Africa are struggling to cope not only with the absence of their young family members through urban or transnational migration, but also with problems associated with ageing populations and diseases such as HIV/AIDS. Further new research agendas are being prompted by the globalization of family life to enhance our understanding of changing generational and network-based ties across different nation states (Levitt 2001; Phillipson 2007).

Migration and the resulting distances from kin and community can place both conjugal and intergenerational ties under tremendous strain. With little support from extended kin, migrant couples are more dependent on their own emotional and material resources. Globalization can also prompt intergenerational tensions through the disruption of traditional patterns of care giving, with older women in particular, usually involved in both giving and receiving. In Mexico – as in many Latin-American countries – many older adults live alone as a result of the migration of one or more of their relatives, mostly to the USA (Rodriguez 2009). They might not see these relatives for long periods, even though they often depend on them financially. While studies of older people have tended to focus on care delivered in distinct localities, research on transnational communities is now increasingly emphasizing the possibilities of sustaining support across wide geographical distances. Gerontology research assumptions that care-giving requires closeness have been challenged (Baldassar 2007:276). A variety of supportive ties are maintained by migrants in practical, moral, financial, personal and emotional ways (Chambers et al. 2009). However, a lack of research on this issue means that we still know little about transnational recip-rocal care-giving practices among dispersed families.

The sparse amount of research undertaken so far indicates that migrants provide support to relatives in their first homeland in relation to their own economic circumstances and in keeping with the negotiated commitments shaped by family histories and per-sonal relationships (Baldassar 2007). Intergenerational family ties are often involved in the sponsoring of migrants' decisions to journey to another country, indicating that intergenerational support is not just one-way. Parents and other kin may have provided advice and assistance with the financial outlay of their child's emigration and the long-term or temporary care of dependent children left behind. In a study of Jamaican families, the care of children whose mothers travel to find work was undertaken by grandmothers (Bauer and Thompson 2006). Transnational care-giving practices are also determined by a sense of duty to provide care which, in turn, is shaped by expectations relating to cultural traditions about social and family obligations. For example, research on first-generation Italian migrants to Australia shows that the obligation to offer care, through remittances, to ageing parents in Italy was often intensified through their decision to remain permanently in Australia, rather than lessened (Baldassar 2007). Other types of transnational care among the Italian family net-works, in the form of emotional and practical support through new communication technologies, tended to be more mutual.

A study of first-generation Bangladeshi women aged thirty-five to fifty-five in Tower Hamlets, London, revealed that 71 per cent of women had a mother alive in Bangladesh (Phillipson et al. 2003). Many expressed difficulties associated with the pressure to give assistance to their mothers despite their own problematic financial situations. Migrants face many challenges in assisting, from a distance, ageing and frail parents left behind in their first homeland. Italian migrants to Australia between the 1950s and 1990s felt anxieties and guilt associated with the difficult attempt to support parents in Italy who were suffering from illnesses such as dementia (Baldassar 2007). In some cases, grandparents emigrate to join their children in the West as a way of addressing their need for support in old age and/or to provide help with childcare to allow the mother to gain employment (King and Vullnetari 2006).

The values of materialism, consumerism and individualism are commonly associated with modernity, globalization and 'the West'. They play a central role for families who have migrated through professional aspirations. For example, Indians are a fast-growing immigrant group in the United States who face the challenges of caring for and sustaining intimate ties with elder parents while parents remain in India or follow their children to America to live in their children's homes. Research by Sarah Lamb (2007) demonstrates that, across India and North America, migration is generating important questions about the proper social–moral relationship between individuals, families and the state. 'Indian' identity has been governed by a system of life-long intergenerational reciprocity and intimacy. Close multi-generational families involve the care of ageing parents by adult children through values of obligation, respect and affection for parents. This system is characterized by households containing several generations. However, now that kin live all over the world, these kinds of values are being undermined by trends associated with western individualism: the decline in extended family forms, demands for gender and age egalitarianism, and the allure of consumerism and material wealth.

Most Indians who migrated to the USA from the mid-1960s[1] travelled as professionals with preferred occupational skills or as students. As this young population aged, many brought ageing parents from India to the USA in response to parents' demands. In 'traditional' Indian society, elders are respected in the society as a whole, not just by their immediate family (Lamb 2000). After arrival in the USA, Indian elders often complain of being neglected by their children who lack time to be with them. This reflects a dilemma being faced across western migrant nations such as the USA, UK and Australia: people seek wealth and yet find little time for intimacy and care. Nursing homes come to provide an important avenue of caring for ailing elderly parents. Given the nature of their work, and the fast pace of life in the USA, daughters-in-law are not regularly available to do the domestic chores expected of them in India.

Paradoxically, senior Indians are responsible for their professional children's material aspirations and success, having ensured they gained the qualifications to migrate. Through their children, parents gain prestige and expect to share in their children's prosperity, which they themselves instigated. Nevertheless, most Indian American seniors believe that the pursuit of material wealth obstructs intimate intergenerational relationships. Lamb (2007) cites one woman who complained that her children have a better life in the USA as professionals, yet she and her husband were forced to live in an apartment alone, next door to their younger son, who apparently seldom visited her. She speculated whether they would be poorer yet happier and a closer-knit family if they had stayed in India. The children are conscious of the irony that their parents seek prestige through their offspring yet the children are unable to care for their parents in the manner expected.

Contrasting with the Indian example in the USA, Kanwal Mand (2008) examines the predicaments resulting from widowhood, separation and divorce amongst transnational Sikh women. She describes the social embarrassment and family tensions arising from a reversal of traditional kinship norms when an elderly widow is forced to take up residence with her married daughter's family rather than her son's. In the North Indian kinship system, senior women are expected to rely on their sons for support in their old age, and not on their married daughters. Indeed, older women are the normal heirs to the parental estate. But among migrant families, far away from their homeland, such customs cannot always be adhered to. In the case studied by Mand, even the woman's unpaid duties as grandmother, enabling her daughter to go out to work, and the affection of her grandchildren, cannot make up for her damaged self-worth. However, Mand (2008) also shows that, for Sikh women who are 'twin-migrants' – immigrants from Tanzania to the UK – migration can be liberating if faced with widowhood, separation or divorce. It can be a means for women to escape the unfavourable mark and dependency of widowhood, difficult in-laws or bad marriages, or a means by which to obscure socially disapproved outlets from such marriages, such as through long-term separation (without divorce).

These kinds of examples indicate that traditions of care for elderly family members can be strict and constraining for women in certain cultures. However, in rapidly modernizing societies, the tensions between familial tradition and modernity are leading younger women and their spouses to find novel ways of dealing with care. In contemporary Taiwan, a form of paid care work is used to maintain patrilineal[2] intergenerational ties alongside the shift to a nuclear family form to resolve the tensions of the old and the new (Lan 2003). Taiwanese family tradition demands that sons return the debt of their parents' costs of bearing and raising children. Married sons are obliged to live with and care for their ageing parents, but the tasks are expected to be carried out by his wife. Yet in contemporary Taiwan, the conjugal, nuclear form of the family has become the norm, with young couples expecting to live separately from their parents. While 60 per cent of households are nuclear, one-third of households contain three generations. The relationship between mother-in-law and daughter-in-law, shaped by the Chinese tradition of filial[3] piety and patriarchal authority, leads to increasing tensions and challenges for daughters-in-law who may have demanding full-time jobs.

The rate of labour participation among educated young women in contemporary Taiwan is high, in response to a 1980s boom in the service sector. Dual-income households are commonplace, with rising housing prices and cost of living. Many wives are therefore frustrated by the unequal division of filial labour between themselves and their husbands and are addressing the problem of serving their duties to parents-in-law by hiring Asian nannies and maids (Lan 2003). A popular arrangement for the care of the elderly in Taiwan is now to draw on a migrant labour force that is paid less than half the wage of a local care-giver and can provide live-in service. This sub-contracting of filial duty to address what is now viewed as an unfair gendered burden involves hiring a Filipina maid who becomes a surrogate carer. A transfer chain of 'filial kin work' is thereby practised as a form of care work to maintain patrilineal intergenerational ties (Lan 2003). A gradual decline of parental authority is evident in Taiwan, with the hierarchical concept of 'serving' being gradually replaced by the term 'caring'. The social norms of filial piety are balanced against the desire for privacy and autonomy among young couples. Couples are now finding ways of reaching a compromise on the demands of family tradition by making other arrangements, such as living in different apartments in the same building, living apart but having meals together, or making regular visits and hiring care workers.

Recent economic development and socio-cultural changes in China have made it increasingly difficult for families to provide eldercare. Institutional care has therefore been promoted by the state to meet older adults' long-term care needs. However, a recent study found a lack of willingness among older adults to live in long-term care institutions in urban and rural areas (Chou 2010). A number of factors led to a reluctance by rural and urban older people to consider living in eldercare institutions. Most believed such a move would undermine family harmony, filial piety, and beliefs and practices about raising children and eldercare. They also had little knowledge about eldercare institutions.

Conclusions

This chapter has shown that age is a significant mediating factor within family and wider relationships. 'Ageing populations' in western nations raise crucial issues about caring and obligation within the family and intergenerational relations, which, in turn, correspond with political and economic processes. The chapter has identified a number of misconceptions about ageing relatives and intergenerational ties. The first is that older people are a uniform group. This chapter shows that, in western societies, older people are now a much more varied group in terms of different birth cohorts, expectations of different social classes and values (Chambers et al. 2009). Differences in experiences of ageing are determined by a number of factors including gender, sexual orientation, location, migration and economic resources.

Notwithstanding the role of traditional kin in providing child-and eldercare, it is likely that in the future, long-lasting marriage and kin ties may be only one of many ways in which intimate relationships are sustained in older age. Increasingly diverse and fluid family-like practices among older people are likely to characterize future experiences of ageing (Chambers et al. 2009). The significance of this diversity reiterates a major theme across the book as a whole. In particular, the likely rise in childless couples and in single-person households among future ageing cohorts means that new social ties, such as friendship, will become increasingly important. Research is needed to understand the implications of the potential diversity in the experiences and structures of ageing (Dykstra 2006; Dykstra and Hagestad 2007). The partnership experiences of older people from minority ethnic groups with their own distinct family practices have been under-researched. Research about older non-heterosexual men's and women's needs also remain limited.

A second misconception is found in the persistent social stereotypes of older people as unproductive, infirm and dependent, whilst the reverse is often the case. In western societies, many older people retain independence throughout their lives. They often remain major players in family life and in wider society through voluntary work or by remaining in paid work well into later life. Thus, the 'culture of decline' associated with older family members needs to be challenged in research on the sociology of ageing and the sociology of family.

A third and related common fallacy is that older people are a liability to younger family members and the state. Notwithstanding comprehensive welfare systems, older generations have continued to distribute resources to their own children as well as to grandchildren (Hoff and Tesch-Romer 2007). Much research on grandparenting in the last two decades, particularly in the USA, indicates a growing appreciation of the considerable amount of material and care-giving resources grandparents offer young families (Minkler 1999; Goodman and Silverstein 2001). Across the world, grandparents supply vital childcare, allowing mothers to enter paid work. Nevertheless, women tend to be significantly worse off after retirement than men. They tend to be poorer, have access to fewer resources from the state, and yet live longer. Several salient issues concerning population ageing, which have a direct bearing on family life, need to be addressed by governments in formulating national ageing policies. These issues include the feminization of ageing; equity and sustainability of welfare policies on care giving; and the challenge of using the older population as a *resource* rather than viewing them only as a *burden* (Hock Guan 2008).

A fourth issue highlighted by this chapter is that rising migration and mobility, both geographical and social, are now raising substantial questions for sociologists, especially in relation to the political economy of informal and formal care. The transnational dimensions of family life need to be taken into account, given that migration is placing major constraints on the provision of care by close family members. While studies of older people have usually focused on care delivered in defined communities and localities, research on transnational communities highlights the possibilities of keeping support going across considerable geographical distances (Baldassar 2007:276). Importantly, Pat Chambers and colleagues (2009:96) point out that the processes associated with migration may lead to a new form of ageism in the twenty-first century. They argue that, marginalized from key support services as well as dominant social and cultural institutions, older migrants may represent an 'urban underclass'. The following chapter picks up on this theme of migration and highlights its importance for understanding the global features of family life. It looks at the impact of globalization and migration on family life in further depth by addressing the range of challenges facing families as a result of transnational marriages and the global movement of labour with a focus on care workers.

6 Globalization, Migration and Intimate Relations

The growing geographical distances between individuals' natal home and marital home are a major feature of globalization. The term 'globalization' refers to those processes and institutions that link together individuals and groups across different regions and nation states. Scholars have tended to study this process in terms of the transnational movement of capital, state and market mechanisms, and new technologies (Robertson 1992; Taylor et al. 2002). Yet a focus on money, markets and flows of male labour has meant less attention paid to women and families, even though they are centrally involved in labour flows (Hochschild 2000). In this chapter, globalization is approached by examining the two key processes of marriage migration and female labour migration. These are analysed through a series of case-study examples to understand how they interconnect with, support and are affected by wider global practices.

Despite its influence, the individualization thesis (addressed in chapter 2) foregrounds a particular western version of intimacy and family life which does not necessarily concur with familial experiences in many other parts of the world. In many regions, marriage is founded on a *contract* between two families, not on romance, agency and choice. It often involves a broker, economic exchange and the transfer of the daughter across great distances. Across regions such as parts of Asia, individual and family aspirations for marriage are tightly connected with social mobility. Another form of contract which involves a migration of family members has been prompted by a deficit in care in western nations and a deficit in resources among families in developing nations. Individual family members travel to the West to find employment as nurses, domestic workers and nannies. They send money back home for their family, leaving their children behind to be cared for by kin.

This chapter examines the strategies of matchmaking involving migration and labour, the transfer of resources brought about through marriage, and women's migration and domestic work. It demonstrates that local and international marriage and labour markets are linked processes mediated by local practices and customs of kinship and marriage. The topics of transnational arranged marriages, including bride price and dowry payments, female migration of care workers, mail-order brides and the global dimensions of internet-dating, are addressed here. In the current climate of liberalization and globalization, bride wealth, dowries and the conspicuous display of weddings are forms of marriage payments that appear to be on the increase rather than declining (Palriwala 2003; Palriwala and Uberoi 2008). Bride price in China and the dowry system in India have grown considerably in recent years (Palriwala 2003).

Through a range of specific examples, the chapter foregrounds the importance of interrogating the connection between the *public* and *private* spheres of society – that is between *politics/economics* and *intimacy* – for an understanding of the way that intimacy and family practices cross these boundaries. Commercially arranged marriages and care work migration are not only evidence of transnational flows of intimacy and care. They are also indicators that intimacy is being used to manage these public/private boundaries on a global scale. The 'intimate politics of globalization' is a term that highlights this interconnection between sex, family, intimacy, the private and the personal and macro-socio-economic issues of labour, capital and populations (Cole and Durham 2007:19). Differences in marriage and kin customs between countries are compared in this chapter through case studies, to provide comparative distinctions between and parallels across regions.

Gendered migration patterns

Until recently, the typical migrant was assumed to be male, with women participating in migration as dependants associated with men's movement through family reunification. Between the 1950s and 1970s, most migrants from Turkey, Greece and North Africa to northern Europe were men. Married women were consistently excluded from academic studies of migration since the economic function and agency of marriage migrants was assumed to be inconsequential. However, by the 1990s women were taking the place of men in patterns of migration, by migrating to the USA, Canada, Sweden, the UK, Argentina and Israel in significant numbers. By 2000, women and girls formed almost 49 per cent of legal and illegal global migrants (Ehrenreich and Hochschild 2003:5). Among early studies that included women in their focus on male migration of the 1990s, is Leela Gulati's (1993) study of the impact of male migration to West Asia on women in the Indian state of Kerala. Gulati noted the challenges facing women who were forced to cope alone with a new family, during long periods of separation from their husbands to whom they had been married for just a few weeks.

The omission of women's migration in past studies led to two problems. First, marriage migration was largely ignored until recently. Second, the routine underestimation of the value of women's work and their careers relative to men's, and the implied model of male breadwinner / female homemaker lessened our understanding of the links between marriage, family and economic migration. Although information on illegal migrants is unreliable and many developing nations lack statistical data on migrating labour in general, scholars have begun to identify a 'feminization of labour' as a clear trend (Castles and Miller 1998; Momsen 1999; Ehrenrich 2002). Importantly, in some countries such as the Philippines and Sri Lanka, women now constitute over half the migrating population (Ehrenreich 2002). In specific migrating categories, such as domestic workers, care-givers, sex workers and family members, women massively dominate (Zlotnik 2003). The current global traffic in nannies, domestic workers, wives and sex workers has dented the view that women typically follow men who migrate in search of work, and has led to what scholars call a 'feminization of migration', particularly in Asia (Ehrenreich and Hochschild 2003; Cole and Durham 2007:12).

Globalization, migration and family care

Changes in marriage and family structures and the growth in women's employment have led to a shortage of labour time to meet the demand for domestic care work. Employers are demanding more flexible labour forces (Houston 2005). This lack of time and labour to undertake childcare, care of the elderly and the daily chores associated with domestic work is referred to as a 'care deficit' (Hochschild 1995). The pressures and burdens on family life associated with the demand for care workers are becoming globalized (Gambles et al.

2006). The deficit in care work is being filled by an intra-and transnational migration of female domestic workers from poorer regions. This crisis of global care has been triggered by several interconnected factors. The erosion of the male breadwinner wage, the rising employment of women, a fragmentation of extended kinship networks and the global reduction in state provision of care are among factors that have contributed to the increased burden on working-age parents in supporting younger and older dependants.

Many middle-class and western married women who work long hours for longer periods of their lives sustain their careers by handing over the domestic work and/or care of their children to women from developing countries (Hochschild 2003a). Moreover, a significant and growing minority of households in western nations are made up of couples where both partners have well-paid, demanding careers in administrative, professional or managerial occupations. For example, between 10 and 20 per cent of all couples in the United States, Canada and the United Kingdom comprise dual-career households (Hardill 2002). These dual-income couples are increasingly dependent on paid care and/or domestic work which involve global exchanges. The globalization of women's work has been driven by the failure of western governments to address the needs generated by women's entry into the workforce. It is a particular kind of work which is sometimes referred to as 'affective labour' since it entails service work in the intimate context of families through the physical and emotional care not only of children but also of adult family members. As mothers, women from developing countries are motivated to seek labour as carers of the children of wealthy families in order to support their own children back home. The growing migration of millions of women from poor to wealthy regions has a critical impact on the families left behind. Women migrate from countries such as the Philippines, Sri Lanka and India to service the needs of affluent western families in regions such as Saudi Arabia, the USA and Europe, as maids, nannies, nurses, sex workers and contract brides (Ehrenreich and Hochschild 2003).

The countries most affected by the export of care labour include Sri Lanka, the Philippines, Bangladesh and Mexico. These countries are referred to in the following discussion. Several governments of these developing countries have been obliged to deal with their foreign debt and unemployment by attracting western strong currency. They have therefore created migration programmes to export their labour to western nations and bring wages back home. As migrant women are viewed as more reliable at returning their earnings to their families than male counterparts, many governments actively encourage women to migrate in search of domestic work as government policy (Sassen 2003). Women frequently send their families over half their wages, which has a positive bearing not only on the lives of their children but also on members of the wider family and kinship network. For example, one of the most extensive campaigns for exporting women's labour is in the Philippines. Foreign debt and unemployment made the export of labour overseas appealing, with Filipino workers sending over $1 billion home a year. Thailand, Sri Lanka and Bangladesh also have labour-export programmes. The Sri Lankan government offers domestic training to potential female migrants by teaching them to use western-style domestic appliances, from microwaves to washing machines (Sassen 2003).

Research on migrant women carers is recent and remains sparse. However, since the 1990s, certain key patterns have begun to be revealed. Female migrants from countries such as the Philippines and Mexico are typically better educated than male migrants, with school or college diplomas, and have previously been employed back home in low-paid but professional jobs (Momsen 1999:10; Parrenas 2001). Men and women are highly motivated to migrate in search of employment. Featured high among motivating factors are the inequalities between western hard currencies and Third World soft currencies, high local unemployment, and a decline in public services such as health care and food subsidies for the poor. By undertaking difficult but less skilled work abroad as childcarers, domestics and care-service workers, women can earn much more than professional employees in their own countries. They are able to send home funds for their families and can even build savings to start a business. For example, a Filipina domestic in Hong Kong can receive fifteen times the amount she would earn as a school teacher in the Philippines (Ehrenreich and Hochschild 2003).

In contrast to factory work, where labourers gather together in large numbers, the types of work conducted by migrant women are often less visible and socially isolating. Nannies and maids typically work behind closed doors in the private domestic sphere of other people's families. The issue of race may also be a factor causing the invisibility of female migrant labour since it involves women who are addressed as 'non-white' ethnic minorities in western nations and who are subject to racism and regularly discounted: Algerians in France, Mexicans in the United States and Asians in Britain. Moreover, the western culture of individualism discourages middle-class career women from admitting that they use migrant labour. Among the time-deprived upper middle classes of the West, servants are no longer on display. They tend to be kept in the background to give the impression of a career woman capable of juggling domestic duties, career and home dinner parties (Ehrenreich and Hochschild 2003).

The decision by mothers to move to a new country raises important questions about the kinds of relationships maintained between migrating members and their families left behind. This has led to disruptions in traditional customs of family care in poorer, developing countries, with children and older family members often being isolated and feeling neglected. However, as yet, researchers are still assessing the costs of migrating women to their families, their children and their wider communities. The reciprocal exchanges that bind households together are often strained, and new arrangements to sustain those relationships are called for. For instance, women often have to live apart from their own children for over ten years, forced to leave their care to grandmothers, sisters and sisters-in-law (Ehrenreich and Hochschild 2003).

Maintaining local dependencies becomes a challenge for migrant workers. There is a growing literature describing the difficult reallocation of family roles when married women migrate for work, leaving husbands and children behind (Gamburd 2002; Parrenas 2006). In developing countries where there is no welfare pension for elderly members of society, the tradition of being cared for by one's daughter as a reward for motherhood ensures security in old age for women. Senescence is a term that means 'approaching advanced age'. In several regions such as Bengal, for instance, senescence is linked with compassion and made meaningful through care (Lamb 2000). In many non-western societies, life chances are much more constrained by family background, associations and religious and cultural customs and values as well as structural inequalities in education, income and social status. Reciprocal exchanges are therefore fundamental to the stability of extended kin relationships in non-western societies. The reversal of provider–dependant roles and the reinvention of 'joint family' arrangements to support childcare are changes likely to place an extra burden on conjugal and extended kin relationships (see, for example, Gamburd 2002). An important outcome of migration in many cases is the doubling, if not tripling, of the migrant woman's burden as paid worker, parent and wife, and carer for elders.

While research is limited, studies are beginning to show how the migration process, as well as settlement, might be impacting on parent–child relationships. Although some children of migrant mothers may be cared for by affectionate and attentive kin, research indicates that these children are not performing well. Children of migrant workers suffer from the effects of absent mothers. They often become ill more frequently than classmates, their perform-ance in school may suffer, and an increase in delinquency and child suicide has been documented (Hochschild 2003a). The emotional deprivation of these children contrasts with the time, energy and affection given to the children of affluent families in the West by migrant nannies (Hochschild 2003a; Parrenas 2003). Children left behind in the Philippines are a group that has grown significantly since the turn of the last century. Children have reported painful experiences of separation (Parrenas 2005). There is no expectation that they will join their mothers, due to immigration laws, although some of their mothers eventually return to them. However, they are often able to communicate directly with their mothers by cell phone or Skype, or via videoconferencing exchanges (Parrenas 2005). The parents and children in these circumstances learn to develop new, globalized parent–child relationships. Such conditions indicate that studies of parenting and ethnicity need to take account of diverse forms of migration-extended families.

In addition to research on current circumstances, retrospective studies have thrown light on the key issues from a historical perspec-tive. For example, a qualitative study of thirty-one women who joined their mothers in Britain after being left behind in the Caribbean during serial migration between the 1950s and the 1970s reveals the suffering experienced by children from broken attachments and poor subsequent relationships (Arnold 2004). Some daughters believed that their mothers preferred younger children born in Britain. Their psychological distress continued into adulthood. These findings reso-nate with a study of Canadian women and men who experienced this pattern of serial migration from the Caribbean (Smith et al. 2004).[1] In many African countries, children are regularly left with relatives who may be able to offer them improved life chances, or are childless.

Some research, for example on African children who are privately fostered in the UK, indicates that this can lead to difficulties for the children involved (Owen et al. 2006). Children are left behind in the context of serial migration which involves mothers who move to Europe and the USA from Latin America, the Philippines, Eastern Europe and so on, in search of work as domestic workers (Parrenas 2005).

Research on Caribbean migrant families who settled in the UK indicates that 'lateral relationships' of siblings, uncles and aunts are of crucial importance in Caribbean 'transnational families', often more so than conjugal relationships (Chamberlain 1999). Grandmothers and older aunts are also important in Caribbean family life across geographic boundaries, which may reflect the central role of cultural beliefs and cultural practices of sharing responsibility for childrearing (Chamberlain 2003). However, evidence suggests that these patterns are now changing. Grandmothers helped to maintain transnational links between kin and assisted with short-term childcare if they were close to their families. However, grandmothers of 'third-generation' Caribbean families who had settled in the UK were less often involved in childrearing than were previous generations and less well known to their grandchildren (Plaza 2002). Nevertheless, Mary Chamberlain (2003) suggests that, although there may be transgenerational changes taking place, these associations are forming a cultural identity for some Caribbean-origin families and may well survive.

Regarding families who emigrate with children, evidence suggests that the children experience difficulties in settling in their new environments. For example, immigrant children are the fastest-growing category of the US population, originating mainly from Latin America and Asia. In 2008, nearly a quarter of youth aged seventeen and under lived with an immigrant parent, a rise from 15 per cent in 1990. More than 5 million youth now live in households of mixed legal status in the USA, in which one or both parents are unauthorized to live and work in the United States. This exacerbates the uncertainty about the futures of immigrant children with concerns that these are unstable, negative social and family circumstances for the upbringing of children (Tienda and Haskins 2011). Although nearly three-quarters of children who live with undocumented parents are citizens by birth, their status as dependants of unauthorized residents hinders integration prospects during their crucial formative years.

Children with immigrant parents perform less well than those with native-born parents, according to most social indicators. For instance, compared with their third-generation age counterparts, immigrant youth in the USA are more likely to live in poverty, forgo needed medical care, drop out of high school, and experience behavioural problems (Child Trends 2010). Parents' unauthorized status can lead to poverty for children and create difficulties in living arrangements. Unauthorized parents are often too afraid of deportation to claim the public benefits for which their children qualify (Landale et al. 2011). Because many people who migrated to the States since 1970 are unskilled and have low earnings capacity, it is predicted that high rates of youth poverty among children of migrant parents and children of undocumented parents, and a lack of political voice, will be among the problems facing immigrants' children (Tienda and Haskins 2011).

Marriage strategies and mobility

Many academic reactions to transnational marriage are founded on a western concept of romance. However, marriage migration is often an economic transaction, closely interconnected with labour migration, and has a major impact on family life. The range of examples in this section, largely involving migration from China and India to various parts of the world, including the West, demonstrates the patterns and diversity of marriage strategies in a transnational context. Yet, in many societies, marriage presents an important avenue for attaining, strengthening and declaring upward social mobility. The intersection of marriage strategies with mobility and migration is also demonstrated by examples of labour migration that lead to marriage migration. 'Arranged marriage' is a practice prevalent in countries across Asia and, although there are disparities in the region, largely between Southeast Asia and South Asia, marriage is often regarded by academic observers as a business deal that transforms a kinship association into a form of human 'trafficking' (Palriwala and Uberoi 2008).

In societies where marriage transactions take the form of 'bridewealth' or 'bride price', the interpretation of this as commercial matchmaking is more problematic (Blanchet 2008; Davin 2008; Lu 208). Marriage migration reflects not only individual but also family aspirations and strategies (Charsley 2008; Gallo 2008; Kalpagam

2008). Marriage may be perceived as a relatively efficient route for permanent migration, especially for women, given the residential restrictions, the visa and immigration regimes, and citizenship stipulations imposed by many governments (Palriwala and Uberoi 2008:31). In the short and long term, marriage can augment a family's 'social capital' and status (see chapter 9). Marriage migration tends to correspond with the labour migration flows. Thus, women and men may accept spouses who, though otherwise not deemed very eligible, are geographically well located (Fan and Li 2002). Many Filipina contract migrants to Canada who initially migrate as paid workers in the domestic and home care sectors eventually find marriage partners among Canadian men (McKay 2003). Despite women's hopes that marriage will be a route out of unskilled work, part of the attraction for husbands is that Asian brides are, conventionally, 'good' housewives. So the irony is that brides remain engaged in the same care work as before but as unpaid housewives.

The Indian 'dowry system' is linked with transnational marriage migration and with the creation of a global labour force (Biao 2008; Sheel 2008). Dowry payments comprise a fluid fund that can be used by families to finance the migration process directly. Xiang Biao (2008) suggests that dowry payments actually play a substantial role in the reproduction of a flexible and globally competitive Indian information technology (IT) labour force. Her study of Indian male migrants from Kamma and Reddy castes of Andhra Pradesh demonstrates that many men use their dowries to pay for their IT education and subsequent emigration. In turn, their prestige as IT professionals and their higher earnings through migration-linked employment augment their value in the marriage market. They increase the dowries given for their sisters and create a cumulative imitation effect among less prosperous, lower-caste and tribal groups. Biao argues that this highly trained, flexible, relatively cheap and mobile labour, on which mobile international capital relies for profits, is enabled through these kinds of local practices. The exorbitant dowries associated with caste-endogamous[2] marriages and gender hierarchies ensure that women will take on paid and unpaid work to maintain families and, with their IT husbands, take the risks associated with international capital.

Thus, as Biao emphasizes, the gender relations of marriage and migration ultimately subsidize global capital. Even for second-generation immigrants, the cost of a daughter's marriage may be remarkably high. Sheel (2008) demonstrates this in her research on Indian diaspora in British Columbia, Canada. Lavish weddings in the Indian diaspora become aggressive displays of ethnic affluence and assertions of community identity, as well as of status claims within the community. Women of the family tend to take a backseat in the proceedings, while daughters are burdened with the awesome responsibility of upholding family and community honour and a reinvented tradition of gender relations.

Commercially negotiated marriage

A body of work on commercially negotiated marriage across the world is developing. This section offers a range of examples from China, South Asia, Taiwan and Indonesia to illustrate the complexities of and differences between regional customs and practices. 'Arranged marriage' is a convention facilitated by parents and guardians, and usually relies on contacts with wider kin and neighbours or local established matchmakers for recommended matches. By contrast, the western custom of romantic marriage involves choice by the couple themselves. It relies on fluid opportunities for personal interaction and emotional bonding between two partners before marriage, within a 'pure relationship' (see chapter 2). Not surprisingly, the idea of introducing commercial imperatives into spouse selection is abhorrent to western thinking, since it seems to undermine the authenticity of a marital relationship. In China, many Muslim societies, and among certain caste groups in India, the marriage transaction can be interpreted as the 'sale' of the daughter or purchase of a wife, especially if it involves long-distance and transnational, commercially mediated marriages. A wife bought in this way may well be sold on by her husband to another man, into sex work or other forms of slavery. As Palriwala and Uberoi (2008:35) state: 'Indeed, there is only a thin line separating mediated, commercial marriage arrangements, the abduction and "trafficking" of women, and bonded labour.'

Long-distance marriage migration sometimes involves international kinship networks among diasporic populations but is usually organized by commercial intermediaries, which could include newspaper advertisements, introduction agencies and matchmaking services, purpose-specific tour companies and internet dating sites (Palriwala and Uberoi 2008). There are several motives that compel women, men and their families to turn to these commercial facilities.

There may be reduced marriage possibilities in their homeland or region, with fewer partners to choose from. Commercially arranged marriages could be prompted by economic or other disadvantages that cannot be concealed in the local context, or may result from a family's inability to meet the local demands for dowry or bride price as in Taiwan (Lu 2008) and in China (Davin 2008). According to received wisdom, *dowry* in South Asia is a form of enticement or compensation paid in a tight marriage market to the husband and his family for taking on an 'unproductive' woman. Conversely, *bride price* is interpreted as a positive valuation of women's productive capacity and a form of compensation to the woman's family for the loss of her productive labour. Marriage payment is directly related to women's subordinate status in society.

To provide some background to the Indian context, feminist social scientists in India have traced a link between female-averse sex ratios (see chapter 7), low levels of female education and employment, women's disadvantaged property rights and high or enhanced rates of dowry (see Agarwal 1994). Although dowry payments constitute a fluid fund that can be used to finance the migration process directly, women can be vulnerable in such processes. Stories circulate about Indian women who have been deserted immediately after marriage by husbands who use the proceeds of their marriages to emigrate, and of women duped by non-resident bridegrooms. Some of them, in notorious cases, have made a business of marrying local women by collecting the dowries and disappearing soon after. This issue is being addressed by the Ministry of Overseas Indian Affairs to prevent the abuse of women and the exploitation of their families by Indian grooms resident aboard (Palriwala and Uberoi 2008).

The long-term decline in bride price practices in various communities and regions and the increase and expansion of the 'dowry system' are indicative of women's low and declining status in the South Asian context (Srinivas 1984; Miller 1989). China has a notably adverse female-to-male sex ratio, like India (see chapter 7). Chinese society is also influenced by the traditions of patrilocality (the system in which a married couple resides with or near the husband's parents); growing regional economic disparities; a prosperous overseas community; and a tight marriage market. These features are combined with a high female work participation rate in China; the predominance of bride price, the rate of which has increased dramatically as a result of the expansion of the commodity economy; overall economic prosperity;

and the increasing demand for women's non-household labour (Han and Eades 1995). The demand for brides from interior provinces is partly motivated by the inability of poorer men in more developed regions to raise the bride price to acquire local wives (Davin 2008). In order to evade this situation, poorer men in the more prosperous areas 'import' wives. The brides' families may profit from the bride price payment at the time. However, the 'bought' woman who is traded to a distant destination is invariably involved in the marriage of a 'less eligible' man and may find she is worse off, by being socially isolated and with a bad bargain in her husband.

Taking Taiwan as an example, we find that marriage migration has grown rapidly since the 1990s with over a quarter of marriages recorded in 2002 as cross-border marriages between Taiwanese men and women from mainland China or Southeast Asia. The proportions are even higher in areas that have high female-adverse sex ratios (due to the familial preference for sons and female out-migration to urban areas). The traffic in wives in Taiwan is quite separate from the traffic in women for domestic work and for sex work. Marriage brokerage varies considerably, ranging from individual marriage brokers and entrepreneurs to commercial marriage bureaux. The latter include travel, introduction, engagement, marriage ceremonies, visa procurement and so on (Lu 2008). Marriage brokerage can also involve informal arrangements by women who themselves were marriage migrants and want to attract more women to set up a community around them. However, transnational marriage is not just about the commodification of women. The material interests, considerations of social status and search for love and emotional satisfaction are all components that may not be neatly differentiated either for the women concerned or their families (Lu 2008:37).

In certain other contexts, there may be an overlap between long-distance marriage and sex work among recruiting agents. Commercial sexual services and domestic/care services are often the easiest opportunities for employment for migrant women, who operate under severe constraints in accessing education and work prospects. Also, marriage may often be a way of enticing women from poor regions into sex work in distant destinations that would convince their families to part with them. For example, Thérèse Blanchet (2008) describes the abject conditions of Bangladeshi girls exchanged for money as wives in Uttar Pradesh, often to poor or elderly men of a different religion, language and country who expect both the girls' labour and reproductive services. In such cases, the lines seem blurred between forced or slave marriage, purchased wives, bride price marriage and a marriage made doubly oppressive by the combination of distance and 'sale'. Vast marriage distances from the natal home for Chinese, Indonesian, Pakistani, Bangladeshi and Indian brides often entail the loss of the protection of the social and kinship relations normally called upon in spouse selection. A newly married migrant woman may be alienated and vulnerable to abuse in a way comparable to the experiences of the trafficked wife, with little hope of any solution (Abraham 2008; Blanchet 2008; Davin 2008; Lu 2008).

In the case of 'bought' wives, the ties of family reciprocity with the natal family are severed, so the wife's isolation from her natal kin becomes total. This is all the more so in cases where the women suffer the stigma of marrying men from a different religion. Brokered arrangements can resemble trafficking and the entrapment of women. The great distance from the natal home not only means a lack of protection for the women against abuse and violence but also less fear by husbands that their wives will run away. Walking out on long-distance and transnational marriage is made difficult by issues of custody and care for children, in terms of moving them across international borders (Singh 2008). Conversely, Chinese women in long-distance brokered marriages may be lucky and have better access to economic independence due to the growing demand for women's paid labour in the destination areas. They may also have better resources to call on, such as non-government organizations working for women's causes, and higher expectations of good treatment in marriage than their South Asian counterparts. China has, after all, experienced many campaigns to change the face of gender and family relations since the mid twentieth century (Davin 2008). These examples demonstrate that transnational marriage is highly complex, diverse and adapted to the challenges and conditions of regional customs and economic circumstances.

Sustaining cultural traditions in diasporic settings

This section focuses on the way that marriage is used to secure cultural traditions in the context of diasporic communities in western nations. The challenges faced in this context are likely to involve intergenerational tensions generated by the adoption of western-style customs through acculturation, rather than poverty. The practice of marrying within a specific ethnic group ensures the transmission of the community's values and culture to the younger generation. Ethnic communities can only sustain their ethnic identities through community-endogamous marriages, either within the locally settled community or by marriage to partners from the place and community of origin. For South Asian migrants to western nations, marriage ensures a channel of communication with their homeland, a demonstration of obligations to those left behind and a strategy of reproducing community identity in diasporic settings (see Abraham 2008; Charsley 2008; Gallo 2008; Sheel 2008). Experience of racism, fears of loss of tradition, and stereotypes about the lack of 'family' in the host society encourage early male immigrants to seek brides from the home country as a preferable choice of marriage partner. Thus, diasporic communities often assume that these women will be more docile or trusting and that they will sustain the production of community identity in foreign lands (see Sinha-Kerkhoff 2005).

However, intergenerational conflict in spouse selection, as between first and second generation migrants, has increased. Young men and women themselves may prefer a second-generation immigrant as a spouse, from their own community to ensure compatibility, or they may assert the right to select their own partner, western-style, more problematically, from outside the ethnic community. The defiance of the younger generation, especially young women, has been publicized in the media. Many young South Asian women and men actively endorse the practice of arranged marriage. Yet the British immigration service tends to equate arranged marriage with 'forced' marriage and assumes the inevitability of intergenerational conflict on this account (Hall 2002).

Complicated tensions and changes in family relations can often result from endogamous marriages for the migrating spouses and their families. Migrant women may value their escape from the powers and authorities of the domestic domain and social lives left behind, and wish to settle into the ways of the host society. However, they may also wish their family of origin to appreciate that they have fulfilled their obligations to their families back home (Gallo 2008: Mand 2008). They may win the respect of their natal family for organizing migration of their kin, yet might at the same time feel exploited by their families at home or in the diaspora (Rozario 2005). Migrant brides may experience an improved standard of living and economic independence or become vulnerable dependants, isolated and trapped in their new homes, and perhaps victims of domestic violence. The norms of material support and care-giving for children and the elderly are constantly renegotiated in the context of migration, both within the migrant community and vis-à-vis the families left behind (Singh 2008). Individual experiences vary according to factors of caste, class, religion and race.

Internet dating and 'mail-order brides'

The question of women's agency becomes more apparent when examples of mail-order brides and internet matrimonial services are under discussion. As mentioned, the dominant western belief is that love and romance inherently contradict economic and status-enhancing strategies. This can obscure women's agency in marriage migration in public and academic discourses on mail-order brides and online arranged marriages (Palriwala and Uberoi 2008). The internet has become a major tool for arranged marriages online among immigrants to the USA from countries such as India (Adams and Ghose 2003). Popular matrimonial websites in the USA integrate domestic and international marriage markets as they are also recurrently used by families in India searching for eligible men and women in the USA, Canada and the UK and other countries, as well as in India. Matrimonial websites range from conservative, family-directed markets to unorthodox self-directed markets that have more in common with western matchmaking sites. Family-directed matrimonial sites often contain a small photograph of prospective partners yet consistently include detailed information about caste, religion, ethnicity, education and employment, indicating the emphasis placed on these features for a marriage, rather than on physical appearance. Indeed, one site, www.matrimonialonline.net, lists hundreds of 'caste' options, underlining the importance of this factor in partner selection.

The distinctiveness of these internet matrimonial services is their focus on religion and culture. Questions can be asked about which branch of Islam users follow and their prayer habits. Western dating sites usually identify individuals with similar interests and mutual physical attraction. However, this type of use is rare in Indian society and Indian diasporas due to traditional Indian attitudes to the body (Adams and Ghose 2003). The western concept of dating contradicts the traditional Indian notion of sex as something to be encountered only in marriage. Yet complexion is a physical feature often listed on internet matrimonial ads, with 'fair' skin being viewed as positive. Most skin tones are labelled 'wheatish' while a dark complexion tends to be accompanied by an explanation. Matrimonial websites can serve a significant role if socializing with the marriage partner is forbidden before parental consent, and if the social customs for arranging marriage have been disturbed by migration.

The 'mail-order bride' practice appears to be escalating in post-communist economies such as Russia, and Asian regions such as the Philippines. In the context of migration and the globalization of intimacy and marriage, the experiences of 'mail-order brides' and sex workers indicate the blurred boundaries between matchmaking and trafficking. Hundreds of websites advertise mail-order brides from these countries (see Sassen 2003; Johnson 2007; Del Rosario 2008). The growth of commercial marriage brokerage services corresponds with the rise in migrant women seeking a more comfortable life through marriage with a man from a more prosperous background. However, many end up in a vulnerable position in their new home, isolated from their natal kin and familiar environment. Becoming a mail-order bride is assumed to be an economic strategy among poor women who are forced to breach the proper moral and emotional basis of marriage (Del Rosario 2008:3; Constable 2003). The commercial nature of the marriage transaction and pornographic images of 'Asian babes' create negative views. However, Teresita Del Rosario argues that the mail-order bride phenomenon is much more complex, with the blurring of the division between women's exercise of agency, their calculating self-seeking and their exploitation by commercial interests.

Research by Ericka Johnson (2007) on Russian brides supports this claim. She shows that difficult economic conditions in Russia encourage young women to be vulnerable to the aspiration for a better life through marriage to foreign men, mostly from the USA. However, Johnson's (2007) research is unique. She recorded the personal experiences of Russian mail-order brides in their search for mail-order American husbands. The women believed they were active agents since the marriage was not being arranged by their parents. She also questions dominant American mass media representations of Russian mail-order brides as 'victims trapped in horrible marriages with lonely, imbalanced men or as gold diggers looking for economic stability' (2007:1). The women interviewed came from small Russian towns characterized by poverty, high levels of unemployment and economic uncertainty, yet into which new western practices were being introduced from the early 1990s. They were from varied age groups and social classes, and had differing education levels, yet she found that their stories had much in common. The gender imbalance in the population allowed men to pursue the tradition of marrying women in their early twenties, thus bypassing slightly older women. Matchmaking agencies emerged to operate on the global market, with the internet providing new ways to access global clients. From this perspective, the internet can be seen as a liberating tool for Russian women in the search for a husband.

Other examples also question the notion of a lack of agency for the women. A study of Filipina–American internet romances by Del Rosario (2008) found that the Filipina women interviewed were not trying to find a route out of economic hardship. Rather, they were intelligent, educated, professional working women in search of 'romance on a global stage'. Economic structures and inequalities are not the only reasons for the flow of internet-matched brides from the Philippines to North America. Del Rosario emphasizes the importance of what she calls the 'cultural logic of desire': the 'white love' that characterizes the post-colonial Philippines' enduring and deferential association with the USA. The internet opens up an opportunity for romance for Filipinas away from the social pressures and surveillance of their own community. The women feel a sense of control on the internet. Unwanted relationships can be ended by the press of a button. When a match is agreed by a transnational couple, the family and community can be accepted back into the event. A corresponding 'cultural logic of desire' exists among North American men who desire Filipina brides because they signify a shy, physically attractive and domesticated mode of femininity that many men believe can no longer be found in the West (McKay 2003; Del Rosario 2008). This divergence of aspirations may generate problems in the marital relationship at the expense of the migrant wife and may be a reason why women's exercise of agency tends to be ignored.

Nevertheless, there is growing evidence that certain mail-order brides suffer abuse. For example, in the USA, severe domestic violence against mail-order brides has been reported by the Immigration and Naturalization Service. Yet the law deters these women from seeking reparation since they are likely to be detained if they seek redress before they have been married for two years. In Japan, foreign mail-order wives are not protected by full legal status. They are, therefore, vulnerable to abuse by husbands and their husbands' extended families. In the Philippines, most mail-order bride brokers were approved by the government until 1989, when reports of abuse of women by foreign husbands led to a ban. However, these brokers have continued to operate in violation of the law (Sassen 2003). A disturbing number of women and girls are trafficked by smugglers to end up as sex workers, servicing the sexual needs of affluent men in the West. It has been estimated that, in Thailand alone, half a million women out of a population of 60 million are prostitutes, and 1 out of every 20 of these is enslaved.

Conclusions

This chapter has assessed the implications of a globalization of intimate relations and affective care by exploring the intersections between migration and family. Two major aspects of family migration have been identified and examined: the migration of female domestic workers and marriage migration. One of the major features of this globalization of intimate relations is the growing geographical fragmentation of families, generated by the physical distances between individuals' natal and marital homes, and between family homes and place of work. Today's female migration is characterized by emotional or 'affective labour' within a new global economy of care to support the care needs of families in wealthy regions of the world. The dramatic rise in independent female labour migration has made this practice more visible since the early 1990s. The process involves complex global transactions in which women from developing nations leave behind their own families to gain paid employment as nannies, maids and nurses for middle-class families and nursing homes across Europe and the USA.

To identify key ways in which marriage transactions are interconnected with geographical mobility, this chapter has explained that local customs of kinship and marriage in many developing countries entail marriage migration through commercial marriage arrangements. These arrangements run counter to ideas about romantic love in western ideologies about marriage. In many societies, arranged marriage is used as a strategy to enhance a family's material resources and as a route for geographical transfer to a wealthier nation. The Indian 'dowry system' is associated with transnational marriage migration and the creation of a global labour force, with dowry payments often used to finance the cost of migration. Endogamous marriage in diasporic contexts functions to sustain cultural traditions but, as we have seen, can cause tensions between generations and between spouses. The chapter also highlights the growing practice of 'mail-order brides' in nations where women depend on commercial marriage brokerage services on the internet to find prosperous husbands in the West. Evidence of the abuse suffered by South Asian mail-order brides in the USA indicates the level of risk that women face, in their search for marriage and a better life. However, feminist debates about women's agency urge us to look beyond public discourse about mail-order brides at the complex distinctions between women's exercise of independence, their search for love and security and their exploitation by commercial or criminal interests.

It is often assumed that moral boundaries exist between the market and intimate domains, implying that intersections of intimacy and romance with money and economy are harmful and debasing (Bailey 2003). However, this chapter has demonstrated that intimacy is inherently interconnected with economic transactions. Studies of marriage transactions and intimate relationships propose that the conventional separation of public (economic/political) and private (family/intimacy) spheres is misleading (Hochschild 1983; Kakabadase and Kakabadse 2004). They have shown that commercial marriage transactions and the purchase of care by wealthy families are intimate *social* transactions framed as *monetary* transactions. In her study of the economic principles that sustain family relationships, Arlie Hochschild (1989, 1995) highlights the gendered roles assigned to men and women within the affective economy of families, emphasizing the importance of women's 'emotion work'.

In a similar vein, Viviana Zelizer (2005) proposes that the expansion of world markets corresponds with the invasion of *all* spheres of intimate life by financial/social relations. She argues that the idea of a separation between economy and intimacy, based on sentimentality and rationality, cannot be upheld. Zelizer refers to the 'purchase of intimacy' to explain financial exchanges of intimate care and how these combine with meanings given to practices of care and affect. This chapter has shown that 'family' has become one of the most contested dimensions of globalization, through marriage migration, global 'kin work' and the sustaining of transnational intimate ties. Zelizer and Hochschild offer insights into the gendered processes of these global transactions by highlighting how processes of 'emotion work', care and intimate exchange not only cross the boundaries of public/economy and private/intimacy, but are used to regulate them. This theme is fundamental to changing family life and is revisited in the final chapter.

7 Families, Fertility and Populations

Governments have the power to control family lives through population policies. This chapter explores the interconnection between family planning policies and cultural values in influencing the choices that families make about having children. Continuing the global perspective adopted in the previous chapter, this chapter focuses mainly on fertility control in countries beyond the western contours to highlight some of the major ways that families have been affected by policies in the past and present. The next chapter continues the theme of fertility by examining how state and commercial access to reproductive technologies combines with powerful cultural values in influencing decisions about having children. In this chapter, a series of major case-study examples have been selected to reveal a correspondence between women's and children's traditionally low status and the way their bodies and lives are affected by government population policies in relation to wider cultural traditions.

Governments and family planning

Anxieties about high fertility levels among the urban poor often determine government regulation of families. Reducing the number of children per family among impoverished nations is also viewed as a key strategy for economic development by international development organizations such as UNICEF and the World Bank. These organizations expect the benefits of smaller families to be conveyed to societies through education in under-developed and developing regions of the world. The state-led growth of birth control across the world was a major feature of changes in fertility practices in the twentieth century (Therborn 2004). However, this process of family change has been neither gradual nor linear. In some countries *coercion* has been used rather than *education* by governments to ensure that families conform to population policies. An example addressed in this chapter is China's population policy. Introduced in 1979, the 'one-child' policy prohibited the birth of more than one child per family. This principle challenged the preference for sons as a cultural norm and organizing feature of Chinese families for more than 2,000 years. More recently, the government has relaxed the policy slightly by ruling that, if the first child is a girl, the couple can have a second child, but not if the first child is a son.

The preference for sons over daughters is found in many countries across the world. It is most widespread in an arc of countries ranging from East Asia through South Asia to North Africa and the Middle East. Sons are vital in patrilineal societies where ancestral descent is traced through the male line. Sons not only inherit property but can confer honour and status on the family. In certain societies the son's duty, performed by his wife, is to care for his parents in their old age. The threat of a population crisis has led certain nations such as India and China to introduce family planning policies which, when overlaid with patriarchal cultural traditions such as son preference, result in a significant imbalance in the sexes. In regions where son preference and large family size is high, girls often receive inferior care in terms of food allocation and health treatment. The strong preference for sons also can lead to the practice of female foeticide or infanticide.

In contrasting circumstances, governments also attempt to *increase* their population size in response to fears about low fertility rates. Fertility rates that are below replacement levels, such as those currently being experienced in Japan and parts of Europe, are referred to as a 'demographic deficit'. In such instances, a range of government incentives attempt to encourage married couples to have large families. An extreme example of this practice was implemented in Romania between 1966 and 1989 under the Ceausescu regime, whereby all forms of contraception were banned or made unavailable, and mothers were awarded medals for having large numbers of children. Romania's population policy is addressed to demonstrate how repressive reproductive policies come to be included as part of national agendas. The control of women's fertility in Ceausescu's Romania, the 'one-child' policy in China, son preference and the sex composition of families in India, and issues raised by low fertility rates in Europe and Japan are drawn on as cases. As Japan has one of the lowest fertility rates in the world, it is focused on as an example of a demographic deficit nation to highlight factors that have led to this trend, and the effects on wider society. These case studies exemplify the intersection of the state, traditional customs and cultures in shaping family values, ideals and practices connected with reproduction, fertility and family planning.

All governments use ideological strategies as part of family fertility control. Ideas about 'good families' are conveyed through the news and government policy reports, and political rhetoric is conveyed within advertisements about family planning benefits and popular discourses on appropriate family size. These techniques are activated through law and welfare, and through either voluntary or coercive means. International debates about population control in the 1960s and 1970s were divided along geopolitical lines into two groups. In the first group, developed western nations tended to support family planning aimed at regulating what was viewed as a population explosion. In the second group, developing and Third World countries tended to adopt the view that governments had a right to shape their own population policies most relevant to their national situations. At the 1974 World Population Conference in Bucharest, at which these issues were aired, it was officially agreed that women have a crucial role in demographic policies. Romania's interpretation of this accord was to have devastating effects. After the destructive consequences of harsh population policies in countries such Romania and India, detailed in this chapter, the 1994 International Conference on Population and Development (ICPD) in Cairo called for greater emphasis on a full programme of reproductive health that would be less concerned with specific demographic goals (United Nations Population Fund 1999)

Romania's pro-natalist policy under Ceausescu

One of the most repressive pro-natalist policies in the world was experienced by the citizens of Romania between 1966 and 1989 under the reign (1965–89) of the dictator Nicolae Ceausescu. By criminalizing abortion in a country where contraception was unavailable, the government forced women to have babies. Kligman explains that the Ceausescu regime represents an extreme case of political intervention into the most intimate aspects of everyday life: 'state intrusion into the bodies of its citizens' (Kligman 1998). During this period, motherhood was portrayed in official rhetoric as a 'noble patriotic duty'. For example, the state newspaper, *Scinteia*, contained articles extolling the nationalistic virtues of large families. After the fall of the regime in 1989, the world's media reported on the disastrous effects of Romania's strict anti-abortion law passed in 1966.

Following World War II, one of the consequences of socialism in Eastern Europe was accelerated demographic change. Mortality rates dropped, life expectancy increased and birth rates declined in response to growing educational opportunities including adult literacy, improved housing, health care and jobs created for women in the waged sector of the economy. Declining birth rates were viewed as detrimental to the socialist development plans. The decline in Romania's birth rate in the 1950s and 1960s was viewed by the state as a major demographic problem for the nation. Ceausescu's aim was not only to modernize and enhance Romania's economic prosperity, but also to secure political independence from the Soviet Union. However, without the resources to develop a capital-intensive economy, socialist economies such as Romania relied principally on *labour* in the quest for modernization. State policy therefore drew directly on demographic factors to build socialism, which, in turn, directly affected the lives of women (Kligman 1992:366).

To trigger population growth in Romania, Ceausescu signed the decree law in 1966 demanding that each family produce four or more children. Decorations were awarded to women who gave birth to several children, including the orders 'Heroine Mother', 'Maternal Glory' and 'Medal of Maternity' (Kligman 1992:377). A tax was imposed on all adults, male and female, above the age of twenty-five who were 'childless'. This tax was mockingly called the 'celibacy' tax by Romanians (Keil and Andreescu 1999:481). A range of positive incentives were presented to women and their families to increase the birth rate. For each new birth, families were offered subsidies and maternal leave was available. Compared to childless couples, families with children were offered favourable housing and privileged access to rationed goods.

The vigorous enforcement of the law had disastrous consequences for many women who found they no longer had control over their bodies (Kligman 1998). The decree coincided with the discouragement of contraception use and the surveillance of pregnancies to prevent their termination. Apart from condoms, safe and effective contraception was extremely expensive and difficult to obtain. The government was reluctant to devote hard currency to importing substantial quantities of contraceptives. Induced abortions were made illegal for the next twenty-three years. The law was only revoked in December 1989 after the collapse of the regime. Women were therefore faced with illegal abortions as virtually the only method of contraception. They were forced to risk the complications of infection, injury and death associated with the precarious medical treatment of illegal abortion. Those who experienced medical problems were refused emergency medical treatment by the state unless they revealed the names of the illegal abortionists (Keil and Andrecscu 1999). The pro-natalist propaganda campaign was upheld and managed through collusion and threats of punishment (Kligman 1992:381). Fertile women were regularly tested at their place of work, such as factories, to check whether they had conceived and to ensure they would not abort the foetus. Sex education was accelerated and organized nationwide through the 'schools for mothers', 'schools for fathers' and even 'schools for grandparents' (Kligman 1992).

Women were affected in a number of different ways. With no contraception, no sharing of duties with husbands, and few labour-saving devices, employed women were continuing to serve the emotional and caretaking needs of their large and growing families as well as the nation. Contraceptives available on the black market were bought by more wealthy and educated urban women who could afford them and knew where to purchase and how to use them. Factory workers bore the brunt of the pro-natalist policies, both materially and bodily (Kligman 1992:383). Many rural women were pressured by the government to sign contracts to have four children and then worried about what would happen if they could not deliver or if a child died. With poverty widespread, women and their families found it difficult to rear large numbers of children.

By barring women from access to contraception or legal abortions, Ceausescu's pro-natalist policy led to a number of dramatic consequences: illegal abortion, a rise in the death of unwanted babies, a trade in babies for hard currency, child abandonment, infant AIDS and international adoption. By 1989, when the regime fell, reports began to be filed about large numbers of children abandoned in Romanian orphanages and stories of tragic infant AIDS cases and an international traffic in Romanian babies began to reach the international media. Until then, a culture of fear prevented the information from being publicized. While Eastern European nations were associating high birth rates with economic development during this period, this type of pro-natalist ideology was viewed as peculiar by governments and demographers of western nations. By contrast, in western nations at that time, attempts were being made to *reduce* birth rates as a way of improving welfare (Cole and Nydon 1990). As demonstrated, in Romania this pro-natalist response to the needs of economic development placed the family under surveillance, and placed women and children in particularly vulnerable circumstances. Romania's pro-natalist policy may seem an extreme example, but it lies within living memory and important lessons can be learned from the events. Contemporary examples of state policies to decrease populations suggest continuing dramatic and often negative effects of population policies on families in various parts of the world, with the main burden placed on women and also babies.

India's preference for sons

A key challenge facing the Indian government in its attempts to reduce fertility levels is that son preference coincides with high fertility among poorer families who do not have access to new reproductive technologies. In most countries and regions around the world where son preference exists, contraceptive use tends to be low. Family sizes expand if the 'right' number of sons has not yet been achieved. If a couple have five daughters, they are under pressure to keep trying for a son. Although fertility levels are falling faster among urban and educated families in India, the preference for sons continues to be intense, even among wealthy families. India is a country with a pervasive preference for sons, where boys carry on the family bloodline and inherit wealth. By contrast, girls are generally considered to be an economic liability due to the burden of the dowry system and the high cost of weddings, especially in high-caste families. It is deemed to be a humiliation for families if a suitable marriage partner is not found for the daughter at an early age. The girl's virginity is considered crucial for her marriage and to protect the honour of the family. After marriage, the girl becomes a member of her husband's family and her connection with her family of origin is largely severed. For these reasons, the birth of a female child can signify the road to financial hardship for poor families (see Arnold et al. 1998; Borooah and Iyer 2004; Dube et al. 2005; Purewal 2010). Although significant changes in cultural values surrounding marriage and family have taken place across the country, especially in many urban areas, these views remain remarkably dominant.

In a culture that mainly views girls as a burden rather than an asset, women are placed under severe pressure to produce sons. This pressure manifests itself in a number of ways. India has a long-standing family planning programme which emphasizes maternal and child health, and even improvements in the status of women. Despite this, sources indicate that less educated, rural-based families are more likely to have larger numbers of sons (Iyer 2002). Alongside families' efforts to bear sons, a large number of unwanted girls are being born with an unusually high risk of dying young. The UK charity ActionAid (2008) reported that rising numbers of female foetuses are being aborted and baby girls being neglected and left to die, despite the existence of the 1994 Indian law banning gender selection and selective abortion. Questions raised by such findings concern fertility decisions, childhood female mortality rates and how family structures affect the welfare of boys and girls. Female infanticide, child marriages and dowry deaths continue to be part of the experiences of Indian women (Purewal 2010). Economic and social factors contributing to these circumstances include property rights, marriage dowries and gender roles.

During the 1990s, selective abortion became more common among urban, educated families to whom current medical technologies are now easily available (Samuel 1999). Today, more and more couples can afford the medical technology needed to determine the sex of a foetus (George 2006). Most recent reports indicate that the wealthier parts of India are implicated, with parents ordering online home-kits that claim to determine the sex of the foetus. Advocates of pro-sex selective abortion in India claim that this technique helps families to cope with rigid cultural customs, especially the crippling cost of a daughter's dowry and the fact that a daughter will eventually belong to the family of her future husband. They also argue that, given the cultural preference for sons, selective abortion protects women from the insecurities associated with producing too many girls: the shame brought upon the wife, the risk of losing one's husband and the high price of dowries (Sharma et al. 2007:856).

Historically, India was the first country to adopt an official policy to slow population growth, in 1952. A situation shared by many developing countries during that period was India's accelerated population growth prompted by declining death rates and high birth rates. Death rates fell as the country benefited from improved public sanitation, widespread child immunization and expanded medical care. Despite the policies and investments in family planning, the Indian population continued to rise during the 1970s. The aim of reducing birth rates through family planning was held back both by deep-seated traditions favouring larger families and by a lack of resources to extend services to an extensive, mainly rural population. Increasing government concern led to the family planning programme's most contentious period. During the Emergency of 1977 resulting from Indira Gandhi's coup, many states adopted coercive measures together with quota systems that led to the establishment of the infamous sterilization camps. Mrs Gandhi's son, Sanjay Gandhi, instigated a forced sterilization plan in which young boys were bribed with transistor radios to entice them to undergo vasectomies. Between 1976 and 1977, 8.3 million sterilizations, mostly vasectomies, were performed, which was an increase from 2.7 million the year before. The abuses and negative publicity generated by the Emergency compromised the reputation of the government family planning programme, and family planning services were suspended (Sharma et al. 2007).

After the 1994 ICPD in Cairo, the Indian government announced that it was adopting a 'target-free' approach in its population policy to reflect the spirit of the Cairo conference. In reality, this new approach has been applied in different ways across different areas of the country. In some cases, local clinics found it hard to operate without specific quotas, such as the number of women accepting family planning or for condom distribution. Some states, such as Andhra Pradesh, continued to offer incentives such as cash (about US$11), or goods such as transistor radios, for women to agree to sterilization. In the 1998–9 period, 67 percent of women aged twenty-five to twenty-nine in Andhra Pradesh had been sterilized, a remarkably high percentage for women under the age of thirty (Haub and Sharma 2006).

India now has one of the highest levels of child mortality for girls in the world. Son preference affects fertility behaviour and therefore the composition of families in every state of India. According to the national 2001 census, the number of girls fell gradually in the previous twenty years relative to the number of boys (Registrar General 2001). How did this come about? Between 1981 and 2001, middleclass families in India aborted more than 10 million female foetuses in order to ensure male heirs, and over a million homes chose sex determination in pregnancy and selective abortion, leading to 500,000 'missing' girls per year (Sharma et al. 2007:855). Daughters with older sisters face exceptionally high risks. In 2008, the charity Action Aid calculated that 35 million women are 'missing' in India, assumed to be the victims of discrimination, neglect and violence. The move towards smaller families in urban areas, ideally comprised of two children, is exacerbating discrimination against daughters. Fieldwork by ActionAid (2008) also reveals that while boy-only families are on the rise, only 3 per cent of families in Morena and Dhaulpur, 6 per cent in urban Kangra and 2 per cent in Fatehgarh Saheb have daughter-only families. Data from Fatehgarh Saheb indicates that families increasingly stop having babies after one son. The chances of a second child being born are disproportionately higher if the first child is a daughter. ActionAid (2008:21) states: 'Most shocking of all are the figures for high caste urban Punjabis, at just 300 girls for every 1,000 boys.' Despite being illegal, sex determination tests leading to female foeticide are common (Sharma et al. 2007).

Abortion was made lawful in India in 1972 for humanitarian reasons. However, selective abortion of female foetuses is not legal, yet has been recorded in India since the late 1970s when amniocentesis for genetic screening was accessible. Prenatal techniques for sex determination were officially used to facilitate the reduction of genetic defects (Ramanama and Bambawale 1980; Ganatra et al. 2001). By the 1980s, when ultrasound technology was obtainable, the practice became widespread. Establishing the sex of the foetus became the main reason for use of the technology by mainly wealthy women. The introduction of the cheaper, simpler and less invasive ultrasound technique provided access to a larger group of people. The technology became a crucial tool in fulfilling the cultural desire for sons. In 1996, India's government attempted to control the rising pattern of prenatal sex determination and abortion of female foetuses by banning prenatal sex determination. It became illegal to advertise or perform the tests, and fines were to be handed to the woman requesting the abortion and to relatives encouraging it, as well as to doctors performing the task. Surprisingly, ultrasound scanning is now accessible in some of the most isolated rural regions of India. A disturbingly high number of pregnancies are now being terminated as more and more families are able to determine the sex of their offspring (see Guilmoto 2007).

The rising abuse of prenatal testing has prompted a heated debate throughout the country. In 2001, the National Policy for the Empowerment of Women produced a policy framework to eliminate discrimination against and violation of the rights of the female child. It stated that, in addition to social stereotyping and violence against women, the most obvious manifestation of gender disparity is the trend of a continuously declining female ratio in the population in the last few decades.[1] Despite laws prohibiting prenatal sex determination, the continuing rise of sex-selected abortions has prompted the Indian government to impose tougher sentences on those performing the terminations (Sharma et al. 2007; Ramesh 2008).

The practice of female foeticide corresponds with the low status of women in certain parts of Indian society. Women's subordinate status is endorsed by religious beliefs and influenced by poor health and education, their lack of control within the family, their low economic position and lack of power in the public sphere of employment and politics. Islam sanctions polygamy, and enshrined in Hindu faith is the privileging of the male child. Compliance and subservience are valued feminine traits, with the woman being dependent on her father, then husband, then son. The husband and his family often control a woman's reproductive health, and her status in the household tends to be influenced by her success in producing a son. Women who request sex-selective abortions tend to have less autonomy and ineffective decision-making powers in the family home, and are more likely to be living in larger joint families where they are susceptible to the pressure to produce male heirs (ActionAid 2008:12). The decision to abort a female child results from direct and indirect pressures from family, community and medical practitioners (Ganatra et al. 2001:122).

Sources suggest that women who are undergoing multiple sex-selective abortions until they produce a son are experiencing psychological distress (Negro-Vilar 1993). Yet numerous abortions can damage a woman's reproductive health (Ganatra et al. 2001). Whilst abortions are increasingly used to prevent female births, the systematic neglect of girls in poorer communities without access to ultrasound technology is contributing to the country's highly distorted girl-to-boy ratios. In poor rural communities such as Morena and Dhaulpur, deliberately poor post-natal care, such as allowing the umbilical cord to become infected, is being used in desperation by some families as a way to dispose of daughters. Spending money on health care or nutrition for girls is often deemed an unnecessary expense (ActionAid 2008:8)

Health clinics are making substantial profits and pointing out the savings in aborting female foetuses (Sharma et al. 2007:855). They attract poor families who are anxious to avoid exorbitant dowries. Some experts have argued that the reason why the prohibition of sex-determination failed to be implemented was that the ban introduced in 1996 was too idealistic (Sharma et al. 2007:856). The ban ignored the reality facing most families: that son preference is a powerful cultural force. To avoid prosecution, health workers are reluctant to provide written evidence of the procedure. The illegal nature of sex-determination and sex-selective abortions, together with the vast size of the Indian population, has made it difficult to establish the scale of these procedures (Grewal and Kishore 2008). The Indian government has introduced a number of schemes to address the problem of female foeticide and infanticide. Efforts to implement the law banning sex detection and sex-selective abortion have included financial incentives to have daughters and monitoring of pregnant women in areas with very low numbers of girls. However, these schemes have been inadequate (ActionAid 2008:24). None of these attempts address the more fundamental and difficult problem of why daughters are so undesirable to most families. The high reward placed on marriage in India through the dowry system places immense pressure on families with daughters. If these practices remain unchanged, then daughters will continue to represent an economic burden, and remain vulnerable to the clash between government policy and cultural customs.

China's 'one-child' policy

China's government instigated one of the most controversial, yet most successful, fertility declines in demographic history in the 1970s when it became clear that population growth might outstrip China's limited food resources. The government set a stringent target to limit the population to within 1.2 billion by the end of the twentieth century. It addressed this goal by introducing in 1979 the family planning strategy of one-child-per-couple. This family planning programme functions through sterilization and abortion and by imposing fines against 'over-quota' children to fulfil its objectives. This 'one-child' policy has become one of the most talked-about fertility transitions in the world.

As in India, China's pioneering approach to birth control has been undermined from the start by two deeply held cultural values:

son preference and the association of large families with prosperity. The idea of controlling the number of births challenged the ancient cultural tradition that a large family is a blessing, a sign of good fortune. This long-standing tradition contradicted the Marxist ideology of building a utopian socialist state. The only way the government could succeed in implementing its population policy was through a combination of rewards and punishments. Those who have exceeded the one-child restriction have been penalized – some brutally, some leniently, depending on region and local circumstances. Over the decades, penalties have taken two basic forms: punishment of the family as a whole; and punishment of the woman's body. First, married couples who bear more than one child have social benefits reduced or withdrawn and even have pay docked from their wages. Second, women are encouraged or forced to undergo abortions and sterilization.

At the level of demography, this nationwide campaign has been remarkably successful. The policy facilitated a drop in fertility rate from around 6 children per woman in the 1960s to around 1.8 by 2000 (Wu and Walther 2006). While China's 'one-child' policy has been a major achievement at the national level in terms of demographic decline, at the level of personal experience the campaign has been distressing for many families. The 'one-child' policy entailed a series of incentives that affected almost every aspect of people's social and economic lives. It affected families' salaries, food provision, health facilities, employment and education. With no health care system, the mass of the population in the countryside traditionally relied on their male offspring in old age. China was unable to provide a nationwide social security system. Most Chinese families in rural areas therefore refused to believe that having only one child was an advantage to their families. And this was especially the case if the first-born child was a girl. The custom of anticipated care by the male offspring meant that village Party officials had to work hard to enforce the 'one-child' policy. Local enforcement involved forced abortion, the under-registration of female first births, and bribery to obtain permission to have a second birth. Government demands placed on officials conflicted profoundly with the demands of the rural people (Poston et al. 2009).

Once again, women and children have been targeted as the 'problem' and have suffered as a consequence. Women have endured enforced surgery on their reproductive organs and whole families have experienced enforced poverty for breaking the contract of one child per family. In the late 1970s, abortion became a key feature of family planning. Women with unauthorized pregnancies have occasionally been forced to have abortions, particularly during the period of strict enforcement of the family planning policy in the early 1980s. In those provinces where work units were fined if they exceeded their birth quotas, women were frequently pressured into having abortions (Wu and Walther 2006). Research evidence suggests that this varied considerably from village to village. Some women experienced numerous coercive practices, and others none. From 1982, China implemented a family planning policy of IUD (intrauterine device) insertion after the first birth and sterilization after the second birth. Sterilization, which is the most permanent form of contraception, continues to be strongly promoted by China's government. Local family planning workers are expected to impose on couples the contraceptive methods needed to prevent unplanned pregnancies. Given that the government promotion of contraception as a method of family planning is intrusive, a large number of married couples have opted for sterilization. As a consequence, sterilization has come to be one of the main techniques contributing to China's fertility reduction (Liang and Lee 2006).

Today, ideology and persuasion are used by a raft of local leaders, Party officials, family planning works, neighbours and colleagues to make certain that women of reproductive age abide by the regulations of family planning policies. Echoing the events under Romania's Ceausescu regime, women are inspected in factories by family planning workers to ensure that they don't have unplanned pregnancies. At the level of neighbourhoods, elderly women known as the 'Granny Police' make regular home visits to check that women of reproductive age are using contraception. The Granny Police even eavesdrop on young women's private conversations as part of the surveillance. Regular medical checks are required for women who wear IUDs to check they are correctly fitted (Wu and Walther 2006).

Reports began spreading beyond China in the 1980s about the persecution of women and families who failed to conform to the 'one-child' policy. This prompted an outcry of human rights violations from the international community. The Chinese government responded to the increasing pressure inside and outside the country by re-examining this radical 'one-child' policy. A policy adjustment was announced in 1984 to ease the tensions among the population and reduce the corruption of officials. In rural areas, a second birth was allowed, and a third one where special conditions applied. This change implied the end of the 'one-child' policy in the rural parts of China. For example, in Shandong, a policy was instated to allow girl-only families to have a second child, after an interval of at least four years. Within two years, comparable policies were adopted in other provinces for rural citizens (Hao 2003).

Notwithstanding the criticisms, an important consequence of the 'one-child' policy is that China has managed to achieve the status of a demographically developed country in a short period of time. The population control policy has been stabilized and institutionalized. Small family size became established as the norm by the end of the twentieth century in China (Liang and Lee 2006). While many observers argue that the 'one-child' policy has contributed to a change in cultural attitudes, China's philosophy of son preference remains very much alive. Urban couples, in particular, have accepted the 'one-child' policy, but son preference is clearly a major factor that encourages abortions. Some researchers and governments have been so impressed by the success of China's 'one-child' policy that they believe it offers lessons for demographic transitions in developing countries. Others, such as Catholics in the USA and elsewhere, have condemned the policy's system of quotas and the compulsory abortions as a severe infringement of human rights.

Today's ideal Chinese family is composed of one boy and one girl, since boys fulfil the patrilineal line and girls are thought to be more affectionate. However, the two-child, one-son policy now enforced in China means that a family whose only child is a boy cannot have another child, through birth or adoption. If they do, they are given an over-quota fine, which is equivalent to two years' salary. Some parents have their second child removed from them by birth planning officials. This policy has led to a population of 'missing girls' (Croll 2000). 'Missing girls', in China's case, are unregistered girls either living with their parents or unofficially adopted. Given that 120 boys are born for every 100 girls, it is argued that missing girls are likely to be the outcome of gender-selective abortions (Poncz 2007). However, the cause of the gender imbalance statistic could be the significant numbers of girl babies who remain unregistered in order that families can try for another child. Nevertheless, the effects for girls of not being registered can be dramatic, given that non-registration denies them access to a range of welfare, such as health care and schooling. Some parents decide to place their daughters in orphanages in order to try for a son, and the orphanages then usually arrange for the girls to be adopted by families in the USA (see Poston et al. 2006).

Sex preference only influences fertility when the custom is combined with strategies of fertility modification and access to technologies of sex determination and abortion, as in the case of India. Likewise, ultrasound and amniocentesis have made it possible for Chinese parents to detect the sex of the foetus. Sex-selective abortions have been reported in China. Women have undergone abortions if they have discovered that the foetus is female. Experts argue that an imbalance in sex ratios will mean that the nation will face serious social consequences in future years (Poston and Glover 2006). The birth of more boys than girls between 1980 and 2001 has serious implications for China's marriage market, which began to emerge in the year 2000. This demographic shift has led to a dramatic fertility transition. This assessment throws up a number of issues concerning gender and power. Parents are already setting up their own dating agencies for their single sons, and these single sons are being spoiled so much by parents and two sets of grandparents that they are being referred to as 'little Buddhas'.

Concern that the 'one-child' policy is creating an ageing society has led Chinese officials to review the social implications of the law. The system of enforcing the policy is less coercive than it was in the 1980s and early 1990s. For affluent families, the fine may seem inconsequential. For impoverished families, it can lead to the confiscation of their property if payments cannot be met. The fact that affluence can buy babies leads to great resentment. Concessions also now exist for those individuals who remarry to have a further baby if the spouse has none, and for couples with no siblings to have two children. The government acknowledges that the enduring preference for boys and use of ultrasound to predict the child's sex to terminate female foetuses is problematic. Like India, initiatives to encourage families to value girls are being developed by the government by introducing special social and economic benefits for girls (see Branigan 2008; Dowling and Brown 2009).

Demographic deficit in developed nations

The government fear of below-replacement-level fertility is mostly confined to the developed world. Fertility decline is operating in conjunction with rising life expectancies to produce a rapid ageing of the world's population, with Europe and Japan in the lead. Low fertility creates anxiety among governments for three key reasons. First, low fertility produces more retired people than workers, leading to serious anxieties about payment of taxes and social security. The second cause for concern is also associated with the economy, as the number of consumers shrinks. Third, governments are apprehensive about the geopolitical implications of smaller absolute size as a nation. However, there are benefits to low fertility. Lower population density can increase per capita income, quality of life and environmental health, as in Nordic countries. The economic problems linked with low fertility can, therefore, be exaggerated.

Nevertheless, the combined effects of low fertility and high life expectancy in the twenty-first century are generating a major increase in the proportion of people of retirement age and above. Questions concerning the role of the elderly, in areas such as employment and health care rights, social exclusion and the family, are already challenging governments across the world. The national population structure of the UK, in line with most western societies, is ageing rapidly. The combination of falling fertility and increasing longevity is having an impact on family structures and resultant relationships, with the emergence of smaller yet multi-generational families replacing the previous extended family forms. This is occurring at a time when British government policy is placing increasing reliance on families to provide health and social care and support for the growing number of older people. Recent demographic studies suggest that measures which encourage women to combine childbearing with paid employment may stabilize or improve fertility rates. However, the evidence is not conclusive, given that the links between female employment and fertility are complex and context-dependent (Dey 2006).

An example of these complexities, with one of the lowest fertility rates in the world, is Japan, which reached a historic low in 2005 with an average of only 1.25 children per woman. This is significantly lower than the population replacement rate of 2.1 (Organisation for Economic Cooperation and Development 2005). Japan is currently suffering an economic slump, a decline in the number of children, and a surge in the population of single people. Debates now focus on care of the elderly and the impact of loss of demand for goods on the Japanese economy, as well as the shortage of labour. Fewer children and increase in the elderly population are said to be posing a threat to Japan's future. Japan's fertility decline, and the consequential rise in the aged population, has caused alarm among its policy-makers. Japan shares features with other industrialized nations such as Italy, Spain and Korea, and other European countries south of Scandinavia which are undergoing similar declines in population. Despite government measures to reverse the trend, Japan's fertility decline is steadily continuing (Murakami et al. 2008).

In developed societies such as Japan, fertility is a reliable indicator of female welfare. The public interest generated by fertility decline has drawn attention to Japanese women's social circumstances and status. Research is suggesting that the low fertility levels being experienced in Japan and other nations of the developed world may be a result of social pressures rather than freely chosen (see Rosenbluth 2007). Low fertility may reflect how difficult it is for women to combine successful employment with childcare and family commitments. Women are reluctant to give up their role in the labour market for increased childcare responsibilities. They are delaying or forgoing having children in favour of employment. Surprisingly, the rate of women's participation in the labour market in Japan has not steadily accelerated since the end of World War II in the way it has in other developed regions such as North America and Europe. The Japanese labour market has significantly disadvantaged women: large corporate firms traditionally exclude women, and the government has created a regulatory environment that generated inter-firm labour market immobility. More women in Japan are expected to leave the labour force when they have children. When combined with the government's inability to provide effective childcare support, this lack of career opportunities for women has discouraged women from combining employment with bringing up children.

The Japanese government has tried to encourage women to combine careers with family responsibilities by introducing family-friendly policy in the form of the Parental Leave Act in 1995. This policy entitled every employee to take childcare leave to care for children under one year old. Employment Insurance Law was amended so that insured persons who take childcare leave are paid 40 per cent of their wage before leave. Reflecting strong cultural traditions surrounding the gendered nature of childcare, workers who take advantage of childcare leave are overwhelmingly women (Shirahase 2007).

The government sector, with its gender equality in employment policies, is more favourable towards childbearing women. Better fringe benefits related to childbearing from government employment encourage women who work in that sector to stay in their jobs after childbirth, with around 50 per cent staying in their public-sector jobs after bearing their first child (National Institute of Population and Social Security Research 1998; Shirahase 2007). In the private sector, the evidence indicates that the larger the firm, the more unreceptive the environment for childbearing women is, and the less likely it is that women will stay in the workforce after having children. Policy-makers and managers of large firms are realizing the value of employment policies that favour working mothers, so efforts are being made to create family-friendly environments. But the overall patterns shows that large firms are slow to alter mothers' employment behaviour. Overall, the evidence suggests that Japan's low fertility rate corresponds with unfavourable employment opportunities and conditions for women, coupled with family values that favour full-time motherhood.

Conclusions

As this chapter shows, populations are considered at a number of different levels in relation to family dynamics. National population policies may seem statistically abstract yet they are experienced, often in dramatic ways, at the micro-social levels of individuals and families. When superimposed on time-honoured traditions and strong cultural values, government population policies can have dramatic and often unforeseen consequences for families' health and well-being, in particular through women's bodies and the welfare of children (Kligman 1998). The case-study examples in this chapter provide indications of the ways in which family policies, religion and cultural values can impinge on individual human rights.

The failure to realize the connections between population policies and cultural customs, in terms of causes and effects, allows technologies and strategies of governments to have disastrous consequences and yet to appear natural, and their power to seem neutral. The set of events in Romania between 1966 and 1989 is a disturbing example of the way that the state directly impacted on people's lives through population regulation. Pro-natalism was viewed by state planners as the best way to avert labour shortages and enlarge their domestic markets. It also counterbalanced an ageing population and served the armed forces with a supply of young men. However, coercive family planning policies that rely on the impact of organized ideology and state power can have alarming unexpected outcomes.

This chapter has also highlighted the effects on women and families of the cultural value of son preference, in relation to state population policies. In male-preferring societies such as India, the problems generated by fertility policies became obvious in the 1990s, when birth control and parents' ability to discover the sex of embryos generated serious repercussions. In India, the pervasiveness of son preference has affected fertility behaviour through access to sex-determination testing and to sex-selective abortion, thereby generating high levels of selective abortion of female foetuses and neglect of girl babies. Prompted by food shortages to reduce its population, the Chinese government was forced to tackle the cultural custom of son preference that had existed for more than 2,000 years as part of its family planning policy. This cultural norm was expected to be shattered by the 'one-child' policy yet, at the level of family customs and experiences, it created serious complications which impacted on women's bodies, the ratio of boys to girls, and the welfare of girl babies.

8 Families and New Reproductive Technologies

New reproductive technologies (NRTs) introduce new complexities into human relations by blurring the boundaries between the biological and social basis of 'family'. They challenge previously held cultural meanings about kinship by offering new categories of parenthood which bring about new kinds of social relations (Taylor 2005). Alongside sperm donation, recent advances in the biomedical sciences such as in-vitro fertilization (IVF), embryo research and surrogacy have presented moral and practical dilemmas concerning parental rights. Market dynamics influence how these scientific practices are made available and how babies come into or create 'families'. Gay and lesbian couples can purchase the sperm or ova to complete the reproductive process and wealthy infertile individuals and couples can pay surrogate mothers to have their babies. Improvements in biomedical sciences raise questions about women's health, their rights to control their own fertility and the rights of fathers. Many of the moral dilemmas surrounding bioethics have been publicized by religious institutions and the family values lobby. In turn, these public discourses have influenced government policy and circumscribed access to NRT services.

This chapter considers the various social impulses to use NRTs, and their effects, by examining the ways in which they contest previously held notions of kinship and relatedness. It continues the theme, raised in the previous chapter, about the ways in which fertility and family life are constructed or affected by cultural values and government policy. In this chapter, commercial access to the various technologies is also addressed. On the one hand, new reproductive technologies suggest the importance given to biological relatedness in the context of 'blood ties'. Yet ironically, on the other hand, they also have the capacity to subvert this goal, as this chapter shows.

Concepts of biological and social relatedness are discussed by drawing on a range of research and case-study examples from the developed and also developing nations. Beginning with the UK as a western example, the chapter demonstrates the lengths that legal systems go to in order to privilege heterosexual relationships as the basis of creating families, by disregarding or elevating biological parenthood through NRTs. In highly pro-natalist non-western societies, involuntary childlessness can have dramatic negative psychological and social consequences. Yet access to conventional forms of contraception is often circumscribed by religious and cultural customs, as well as poverty. The serious ethical issues associated with NRTs in relation to cultural and religious customs in minority ethnic communities in the West are examined. This is followed by a study of the Middle East as a key example of the way religion has shaped uses of and attitudes towards NRTs. The market issues concerning surrogacy and the commodification of fertility are addressed through a case study of surrogacy in India, complementing the focus on India in the previous two chapters.

Assisted conception and relatedness

New reproductive technologies are often described as 'assisting nature' by assisting the natural process of reproduction, yet they interfere with the 'naturalness' of the reproductive process (Taylor 2005). Assisted reproductive technologies came about in England in 1978 with the birth of the world's first 'test tube baby' through the technique known as in-vitro fertilization (IVF). Since then, developments in NRTs have increased reproductive choice by facilitating men's and women's access to fertility. The only reproductive technologies available to infertile couples during the 1980s were artificial insemination and in-vitro fertilization. A large number of options are now available, typically offered to those with fertility problems and those who wish to avoid passing on inheritable health conditions to their offspring. The scientific, medical, ethical and legal communities have had difficulties in keeping up with the complications posed by these advances involving the introduction of a third party in the reproductive relationship. The term 'third-party-assisted conception' is used to describe the process in which someone other than a sexual/intimate partner provides the gametes[1] or gestation necessary for reproduction (Robertson 1994). Third-party-assisted reproduction includes egg, sperm or embryo donation, as well as surrogate motherhood. The term draws attention to the fact that a third person is introduced into the condition of two-party parenthood. This third person may or may not be known to the recipient couple or individual.

Societal perceptions of motherhood and fatherhood are being challenged by NRTs because such technologies have the potential to introduce a different kind of relationship with kin, which can also involve wider kin relations of the donating relative. These changes to social perceptions are both conceptual and legal. New reproductive technologies can undermine the idea of 'motherhood' as an integrated biological process since, through NRT, it is no longer certain and specified. A woman who donates an egg to help her sister become pregnant is the genetic mother but no longer considered to be the 'real' mother. However, since the donor as biological mother would have a special attachment with the child, concern has arisen that the aunt donating (or even grandmother) might jeopardize the relationship between mother and daughter or sister and sister (Edwards 1999). Thus, the nurturing role of the mother is no longer premised on the *biological* process. It becomes a key element of a *social* process (Strathern 1992). A child could have three biological parents composed of the genetic father, the genetic mother and the gestational mother. The problems arising in defining the child's 'real' father and 'real' mother are discussed below in relation to the complex and fascinating case of the UK's Warnock Committee. The practice of IVF, which allows infertile couples, single women, lesbian couples and mature women to have children, can be interpreted as extending individualization, choice and the project of self in late modernity (Kehily 2010).

Approaches to new reproductive technologies

One of the barriers to understanding the social effects of new reproductive technologies is that they treat social problems as biomedical questions (Thompson 2005). Research in sociology on the effects of NRTs on kinship draws on science and technology studies and feminist approaches. Science and technology studies (STS) examines scientific research and technological innovation in the context of social, political and cultural values. The approach aims to understand the ways in which research and technological innovation affect society, politics and culture. The issues studied include the relationship between science, technological innovations and society, and the developments and risks associated with science and technology. This approach is often combined with feminist approaches for the study of NRTs. Thompson (2005) distinguishes between two phases of feminist theorizing of NRTs. The work in Phase 1 includes radical feminist critiques of infertility and challenges liberal accounts of reproductive technologies. The scholarship in Phase 2 has reclassified the debates by emphasizing women's agency and women's experiences in the process.

Mainstream or liberal western feminist support for biomedical reproductive techniques in Phase 2 is based on the grounds that the technologies offer reproductive choice and freedom for women. By contrast, the radical feminist critiques of Phase 1, from 1979 to the mid-1980s, were founded on anxieties about the extreme medicalization of reproduction. For example, Janice Raymond (1993) argued that these technologies violate the integrity of women's bodies, perpetuate prostitution and international trafficking in women and children, and are a threat to women's basic human rights. A patriarchal and interventionist medical establishment was perceived to be controlling women's bodies. Research in the 1980s indicated that working-class and minority ethnic women were victims of medical experiments, negligence and lack of respect. Feminist writers argued that reproductive medicines were subjecting women to increased surveillance and so they aimed to reclaim natural childbirth for women (Bernard 1974; Donnison 1977; Ehrenreich and English 1978; Kitzinger 1978; Homans 1986). In-vitro fertilization (producing so-called 'test-tube babies') caused the most controversy. Nevertheless, liberal and radical feminists were united in the search for safe, affordable and accessible contraceptives, which form part of 'old' reproductive technologies. Moreover, with forethought, certain radical feminists advocated the subversion of these technologies to undermine compulsory heterosexuality and assist lesbian parenting through self-insemination (see also Mamo 2007).

More overtly political dimensions of feminist research into infertility medical practices addressed the stratification of families by gender, class, race, age and country, and focused on issues such as transnational reproductive politics. These included criticisms of the widespread use of prenatal testing for female foeticide in relation to son preference in South Asian societies, and abuses of sterilization, testing and dumping of contraceptives, and access to family planning and abortion (see chapter 7). From the mid-1980s, a pattern emerged in which most patients were high-paying consumers who were not suffering life-threatening conditions but pursuing life goals. The business of reproductive technologies followed market strategies. However, conflict emerged between the surrogate and biological mothers-to-be regarding their status in relation to the foetus. The payment of poorer women to be surrogate mothers for wealthy, western infertile couples brought class and First World / Third World issues to the fore. Feminists were also drawing attention to the fact that single and lesbian women were being denied access to NRTs by clinics that implicitly or explicitly restricted their services to what they defined as 'proper' families: heterosexual, married couples.

Phase 2, from around 1992, moved beyond the structural-functionalist explanations for gender stratification by endorsing motherhood and women's experiences. Writers now argue for a return to *agency* for infertile women, acknowledging the authenticity of the maternal instinct (Thompson 2005). The focus is now on *relatedness* rather than traditional concepts of kinship, and is being explored from the anthropological and sociological approach of 'the new kinship studies' (Strathern 1992, 2005; Franklin 1997; Franklin and Ragone 1998; Franklin and McKinnon 2002; Konrad 2005; Thompson 2005). Thus, these studies emphasize the interconnection of biological reproduction and the personal, political and technological meanings of reproduction by drawing on science and technology studies, feminist theory, history and ethnography.

This recent approach allows us to explore the *meanings* that people attach to transfers of 'substance' such as eggs and sperm in specific historical circumstances. It also provides a model for discussing the ways in which bodies and the idea of 'belonging' are classified and used in the clinic, by the state and by other institutions that mediate transfers of bodily substance, and for discussing the implications of these processes (Weston 2001). The work in Phase 2 is also marked by a moral ambivalence, especially concerning the issue of involuntary childlessness among the poor as well as the rich (May 1995), and also the remarkable degree of agency exercised by infertile women patients (Marsh and Ronner 1996). However, the approaches of Phase 2 have been criticized for failing to focus sufficiently on infertility, stratification and difference in order to highlight injustices and inequalities of the practices of NRTs. Importantly, the work in Phase 2 has brought work on infertility and NRTs into the framework of transnational politics of reproduction. For example, in non-western pro-natalist societies, infertility deprives women of status. In western liberal democracies, procreative tourism is practised as a solution to infertility.

Donor insemination and the regulation of families

Donor Insemination (DI) entails the insemination of a fertile woman with sperm donated by a stranger. Its use in the UK was first recorded in the 1940s. This technique requires no sophisticated technology or medical supervision. Many women self-inseminate with no medical assistance (Saffron 2001). Given the simplicity and relatively high success rate of this method, it is popular among the medical profession and recipients. Nevertheless, religious, governmental and medical statements indicate that DI provokes profound socio-cultural anxieties (Haimes 1998). Anxieties centre on issues about the technique, the repercussions for children born through its use, and who should use it. In terms of the technique, the moral concerns about masturbation have been about whether the technique is equivalent to adultery if used with a married couple, and whether women might inseminate without the knowledge of their partner, rendering them 'unfaithful'. Anxieties about who should be able to use DI have been generated by the potential for single women and lesbian couples to create fatherless families through its use. Unease about children born of DI involves questions about whether they should be told how they were conceived, whether this may damage their emotional and psychological development, and what they should be told about the donor. There are also concerns that, if donors produce numerous children, the offspring might inadvertently commit incest as adults.

Notwithstanding the publicized concerns about DI, this method became a recognized medical procedure by the early 1980s to address the problem of male infertility in western nations. However, one of the major concerns surrounding this NRT has been legitimacy, particular in relation to the status of fatherhood. Children conceived through donor insemination signify a conscious effort to create a biological link between parent and child. Fatherhood is uncertain and has to be socially established. It is useful to look in some detail at an example of the way governments attempt to uphold particular versions of 'family' in the regulation of DI use. Since NRTs generate problems about the child's 'real' father and 'real' mother, the Warnock Committee was established in the UK to give advice on issues of parenthood. Taking on the recommendations of the Committee, the Human Fertilization and Embryology Act (1990) (henceforth, the 1990 Act) which regulates assisted reproduction in the UK, did not regard the status of *donor* of reproductive resources as an adequate form of relatedness to constitute a *kin* relationship (Strathern 1992). By removing the donor's status as parent, natural parenthood could be removed as a legal definition in confirming or denying one's status of parenthood. However, if the birth experience was seen as primary in defining motherhood (Warnock 1985), then surrogacy could be perceived as undermining motherhood (Haimes 1990). The 1990 Act confirmed that conception can be achieved without heterosexual penetrative sex.

The objective of the Act was to promote heterosexual, nuclear families and particularly the paternal relationship as the primary framework for defining family life. Remarkably, the new complications that it created in distinguishing between genetic and social fatherhood were suppressed by legitimizing *social* fatherhood over *genetic* fatherhood. In the case of sperm donors, the 1990 Act removed genetic fathers' legal and financial responsibilities to any children they might produce and allowed the *social* father to enter his name on the resulting child's birth certificate. Other decisions in the 1990 Act gave donor anonymity, left parents to decide whether or not to inform their children about the circumstance of their birth, and integrally linked the welfare of children born of assisted conception technologies (ACTs) to their need for a father. The idea of the need for a father in all families conveyed the notion of the inferiority of all other family types and gave a clear steer to medical practitioners about who should have access to the ACTs.

The legal category of illegitimacy had been virtually abolished in the Family Law Reform Act 1987 (Fox Harding 1999) and this allowed the 1990 Act to make provision for the mother's male partner to register himself as the child's legal father. Potential harm to donors, recipients of sperm, the resulting children and wider society is reduced by applying heteronormative frameworks and expectations about family and kinship. The legislative and medical frameworks for the provision of DI were concerned with keeping the donor's identity anonymous, controlling the sperm, protecting the *social* father and protecting the integrity of the DI family and the donor's family, based on boundaries drawn around the adult relationship. Although it contradicted the trend to reinforce parental (paternal) relationships in defining family life, this decision conformed to the way family law has traditionally interpreted paternity: blood ties were less important than the marriage contract in defining familial relationships and paternity (Smart 1987). As Catherine Donovan (2006) argues, the regulation of donated sperm through its collection and use is a way of regulating the exchange of sperm across *bodily* and *social* boundaries. The medical framework 'imposes social order on a technique that could otherwise have resulted in social chaos' (Donovan 2006:501). Attempts were also made to regulate self-insemination by legislating that frozen gametes could only be kept and administered by licensed medical practitioners. Donovan (2006) points out that, elsewhere, guidelines were added to the Child Support Act (McDowell 2004) which in effect mean these informal arrangements have no legal validity. The informal donor / biological father remains legally responsible for his children and thus creates, perhaps ironically, 'pretended family' relationships where these may not have existed.

The Warnock Committee's recommendation on the regulation of those families created through the use of the ACTs reveals three ways of defining family: through structure, ideology and genetic relationships (Haimes 1990:167). In the context of gamete and embryo donation, if the structural and ideological features of the family are not contentious, then *genetic* relationships are deemed of least importance. In other words, if the resultant family 'looks right', by recreating the ideal heterosexual nuclear family, then the genetic links are considered not to be an issue and can be ignored. It is only if the structural or ideological features of the resulting family raise concern, as in the case of lesbian parents, that the genetic relationships become significant and questions are raised about the child's need for a (genetic) father.

Increasing unease was generated by the 1990 Act about the potential use of DI to create fatherless families. No condition was made about who should have access to the reproductive technologies, except that the decisions must be guided by the 'best interests of the child'. An Early Day Motion on the Impregnation of Women was produced by Conservative Member of Parliament (MP) Ann Winterton (1989), who was worried that giving access to DI to 'unmarried' women and lesbians 'undermine[s] the status of marriage, corrupt[s] the family unit and leave[s] the ensuing children at grave risk of subsequent harm'. In response, the Act was successfully amended in the 'welfare of the child' clause to oblige doctors to consider the resulting children's need for a father before access is given (S13[5], 1990 Act). In the context of donated gametes, the legislation's intention was to deny children knowledge of their genetic father. This requirement does not appear incongruous because the term 'father' in the clause is to be interpreted as a social or symbolic father. A social or symbolic father is favoured over no father in the case of single heterosexual women or lesbians, and preferred over the revelation of the identity of the genetic father. The idea, then, was to restrict access to DI for single heterosexual women or lesbians because of the lack of the 'social' father (in addition to the lack of a biological father, due to the anonymity of the biological father as donor). As Catherine Donovan (2006) states, the reasoning is determined by a general allegiance to a particular family structure: 'By promoting and constructing normative family structures in which "normal" parental relationships could be assumed to exist, the potential of DI and donated eggs and embryos to disrupt normative understandings of family can be contained' (2006:503).

However, from 2005, donor anonymity in the UK was suspended, so that children born as a result of gamete (sperm, eggs) donation in the UK now have the right to acquire information about their donor's identity when they reach eighteen years of age. This change reflects the fact that family and intimate life emerged as a major political concern in the closing decades of the twentieth century. Donovan (2006) explains that an outcome of changes in family law led to genetic fathers and genetic kin relationships being given greater priority in regulating non-heterosexual families. Donovan (2006:495) argues that 'These changes can be read as attempts to impose a regulatory framework on the apparent social chaos resulting from changes in the ways adults become parents and conduct their intimate lives in Britain.' The changes made to the 1990 Act led to a move away from regulating family life on the basis of the *adult social relationship* towards a focus on the *genetic relationships* that exist between fathers and children. Since this framework is more explicitly applied to families and parental relationships *outside* the heteronormative ideal, it reinforces the continued significance of that relationship as an ideal.

This change coincided with a string of other changes in family law which sought to reinforce the centrality of heterosexual, nuclear family life and first (biological) families for the welfare of children, including the Child Support Act 1990, the Children Act 1989, the

Criminal Justice Act 1991 and the Criminal Justice and Public Order Act 1994. These pieces of legislation promoted parental responsibilities as 'binding', 'determined by biology' and involving 'serious liabilities'. It is argued that the emphasis on biological parental relationships in the Children Act 1989, the Child Support Act 1991 and the Family Law Act 1996 fragments families across several households and makes *biological* relationships the preferred parental and familial relationships (Smart and Neale 1999:174). Fatherhood changed from a relationship with children based on marriage with the children's mother into a direct relationship with children based on genetic links (Smart and Neale 1999:179; see chapter 3). As Richard Collier (1999) has argued, debates about 'the crisis in the family' have been associated with 'the crisis of fatherhood', resulting in family law that prioritizes the reintegration of *biological* fathers into their children's lives. In addition, Collier points out that this shift occurred in tandem with a reorganization of the needs of children and their relationships with their genetic parents. The principle of children's welfare has been reinterpreted as the need of children to stay in contact with (preferably 'involved') fathers (see chapter 3). In the context of reconfiguring 'family', paternal relationships and the welfare of children, the decision in the Human Fertilization and Embryology Act 1990 to require *donor anonymity* stands out as an anomalous one (Donovan 2006).

Views on infertility treatment among the South Asian diasporas

In this section, ethical issues concerning infertility raised by British minority ethnic communities are addressed in order to highlight cultural and religious influences. Research evidence indicates that minority ethnic communities, such as among the British South Asian diaspora, differ from white British communities with regard to the significance attached to childlessness and ideas about the acceptability and suitability of infertility treatments (Culley et al. 2007). Like many societies across the world, British South Asian communities from the Indian subcontinent are highly pro-natalist (Reissman 2000; Bharadwaj 2003; Widge 2005). Although this standpoint is being challenged to some extent by the younger generation in British South Asian communities, mandatory parenthood continues to be a dominant ideology (Culley and Hudson, 2006). Infertility remains highly stigmatized, especially for women, in the South Asian diaspora and can affect wider social relationships dramatically (Jayaram 2004; Culley and Hudson 2006).

A severe shortage of gamete donors, especially egg donors, from 'non-white' ethnic groups causes couples to experience lengthy waiting times for treatment (Golombok and Murray 1999; HFEA 2006). Issues regarding the willingness of South Asian women and men to consider donating or receiving gametes were explored in a significant study of the public understandings of gamete donation among British South Asian communities, comprising British Indian, Bangladeshi and Pakistani communities (Culley and Hudson 2009). All female participants reported parenthood as essential, and childlessness as socially unacceptable. Across all the ethno-religious groups, women confirmed the shame associated with childlessness, the tendency to hold the wife responsible for infertility, and the grave consequences for childless women. Childlessness in marriage is viewed not just as an issue for the couple themselves. Childless couples are usually scrutinized by the community and women experience negative responses, particularly from in-laws. In some cases, it was suggested, the consequences for the relationship could be severe, as indicated by one participant:

> Having a child is very important. Without children in the marriage problems arise. Life is not as nice and pleasant in a childless marriage. Your husband may be OK with it, but your in-laws may not be so kind. They will try to get your husband to remarry in order for him to have children. (Bangladeshi woman, focus group [FG] 3, quoted in Culley and Hudson 2009:253)

Culturally, a child conceived using donated sperm is likely to generate serious problems for the emotional welfare of the social father, for the couple's standing in the community and for any prospective children. A child, especially a male child, is expected to share a genetic link to the wider kin through the blood connection to the father, in order to carry on the 'family line'. Likewise, a man is expected to have a biological association with the child in order for effective fathering to occur. Most participants believed that men are less able to nurture and connect with children if they are not biologically related, as in the case of stepchildren and adopted children. Fatherhood 'appeared to be highly geneticized' (Culley and Hudson 2009:256). Thus, employment of third-party sperm would not provide an appropriate connection of 'substance' to the male and is therefore deemed to be objectionable for most. The need for biological paternity is expressed in terms of tradition, religion and as part of male authority, identity and power, particularly for Muslim women. In Europe and the Middle East, the belief that human life is passed on through males has endured up to the turn of the twentieth century (van Rooij et al. 2004; Inhorn 2005; Culley and Hudson 2009). For many, especially Muslim women, non-conjugal sperm introduced into the married female body corresponded with adultery. Beliefs about gender and reproduction involve perceptions of egg donation as a familial, clinical and asexual process, while semen donation is viewed in an individualistic way with 'dubious sexual connotations' (Haimes 1993).

The women in this study perceived the use of donated eggs to be a more acceptable and involved technique, allowing both parents to have a sense of control over the conception procedure, and for the child to be linked to both parents. The woman would be bonded with the child through gestation and birth, and the father would preserve the necessary genetic connection with the child, ensuring his social connection as father and the maintenance of the family 'line', particularly in the case of male offspring. In the case of using third-party eggs, gestation and birth were viewed by some to bestow a 'blood relation' to the woman and therefore to both parties. Culley and Hudson (2009:258) refer to this as 'embodied motherhood', where the suffering and pain of birth is seen to cement the bond with the foetus/child. However, most of the women in the study had concerns about becoming donors themselves. These hypothetical donors viewed themselves as connected emotionally to the donated egg and as having some parental accountability to it. By contrast, for the South Asian women, donation within families was viewed as contentious because they felt that it could provoke family conflict. They feared that donors may wish to interfere or even wish to claim the child if they believed the child was 'theirs' and was being inadequately cared for. Many women were also concerned about the feelings provoked if a donor-conceived offspring were to contact them later in life. The suspension of donor anonymity in the UK from 2005 results in all donors facing the prospect of future contact by a donor-conceived child. This was regarded as highly awkward since it would reveal an action that contravened traditional cultural boundaries of appropriate conduct.

The introduction of a third party, through technological intervention, was also considered a hindrance. The use of donated gametes in infertility treatment was considered very much as a 'last-resort' treatment by participants since it transgresses many cultural and, in some cases, religious norms. The professed problems facing South Asian women and men who might consider the process of gamete donation differ considerably from those facing white couples. Infertility is generally perceived as a *personal* crisis and treatment a matter of individual choice in the white community, whereas the British South Asian women reported a further pressure involving more overt *community* demands to fulfil a marriage by producing children. Donated eggs were viewed as part of a medical treatment, while using donated sperm maintained sexual connotations. Women's overt anxieties were articulated through the distinctive attributes of their culture, including religion and gender roles in South Asian communities (Culley and Hudson 2009).

Donor technologies in the Muslim Middle East

Around the world, infertility is a serious problem, with 8 to14 per cent of couples affected (Bentley and Mascie-Taylor 2000). Male infertility comprises at least half of infertility cases globally and is generally more difficult to treat. Yet infertility is, ironically, considered to be a 'woman's problem' (Inhorn 2007). The role of male infertility is greatly underestimated and concealed in several societies. As a consequence, women usually bear the blame for the reproductive failing, which leads not only to anxiety, grief, fear and social stigma but also to marital penalties of divorce, abuse, polygamous remarriage or abandonment (Van Balen and Inhorn 2002). Thus, infertility can make a woman physically and economically vulnerable. Infertility is beginning to be acknowledged as part of the global reproductive health agenda, evolving from the 1994 United Nations International Conference on Population and Development in Cairo. However, so far there are no guidelines on how to apply the objective of prevention and treatment of infertility within concrete strategies. Yet one of the main reasons for people seeking health care in many countries is infertility (Inhorn 2007).

In many non-western countries, alternatives to biological parenthood such as adoption or 'child-free living' are not tolerated as solutions. In response to the problems posed by infertility and widespread adoption restrictions, assisted reproductive technologies (ARTS) have become a global business (Inhorn 2007). These technologies are rarely subsidized for the poor, and are therefore out of reach for most couples in the developing world since they cost from $2,000 per cycle. and up to $20,000 per cycle in the USA. Moral concerns about ARTS are also complex in societies such as the Muslim Middle East, for example Lebanon, Egypt and Iran. There are major differences in approach between the Sunni and Shi'a sects of Islam towards third-party gamete donation. Eight years after the 1978 birth of the first test-tube baby in the UK, IVF clinics began to open in the Middle East, with the first in Cairo. By the 1990s, IVF clinics were available across the twenty-two nations of the Middle East, including the small nations of Qatar and Bahrain. Extensive anxieties and arguments have been generated by these technologies. Religious authorities, physicians, lawyers and social scientists have been debating the appropriateness of ARTS, gamete donation and other new forms of biomedical interventions.

In Egypt, the Sunni Islamic standpoint on ARTS was declared by the first fatwa[2] on medically assisted reproduction. It permits IVF through the use of eggs from the wife with the sperm of her husband and the transfer of the fertilized embryos back to her uterus. Yet no third party can encroach on the marital practices of sex and procreation. This renders a third-party donor unacceptable. These fatwa declarations have, for the most part, been upheld by physicians in the Muslim world, according to a 1997 global survey (Meirow and Schenker 1997). Sperm donation in IVF and all other forms of gamete donation were forbidden on three grounds: the connection with adultery by bringing a third party into the sacred dyad of husband and wife; the prospect of half-sibling incest among the children of anonymous donors; and the uncertainty of kinship, lineage and inheritance in patrilineal societies of the Muslim Middle East. However, Marcia Inhorn (2007) points out that change has occurred for Shi'ite Muslims since the publication of the global survey. Several Shi'ite religious authorities endorse the majority Sunni standpoint that third-party donation should be strictly forbidden. Yet, in the late 1990s, the use of donor technologies was authorized. Ayatollah Khamanei stated that both the donor and the infertile parents, regarding egg and sperm donation, must obey the religious codes about parenting. But the donor child may inherit only from the sperm or egg donor, as the infertile parents are perceived as equivalent to 'adoptive' parents.

For Shi'ite Muslims the circumstances are more complex. As

Shi'ites use a form of individual reasoning known as *ijtihad*, many Shi'ite religious authorities make their own determinations about sperm and egg donation. Key disagreements continue to exist around issues such as whether donation is acceptable at all if donors are unknown; whether the offspring should take the name of the infertile father or the sperm donor; and whether the husband of an infertile woman should assume a provisional marriage with the egg donor and then release her from the marriage immediately after the embryo transfer to avoid adultery. In principle, only single women or widows can accept donor sperm, in order to avoid the charge of adultery. However, single motherhood of a donor child is likely to be socially objectionable in Muslim countries. These moral ambiguities mean that married infertile Shi'ite couples who wish to undertake third-party donation according to religious guidelines have difficulties in adhering to these requirements, particularly in the case of sperm donation. Nonetheless, in the Shi'ite Muslim communities such as Iran and Lebanon, some Shi'ite couples are starting to receive donor gametes and donating their gametes to other infertile couples. For infertile Shi'ite couples who accept the idea of donation, the introduction of donor technologies has been described as a 'marriage saviour', helping to avoid the 'marital and psychological disputes' that may arise if the couple's case is otherwise untreatable (Inhorn 2007).

Ironically, a new solution for male infertility has increased the potential for divorces. Intracytoplasmic sperm injection (ICSI) is a recent form of IVF to overcome male infertility. It allows men with very low semen profiles to produce biological children of their own. The introduction of ICSI in the Middle East in the mid-1990s led to a massive rise in infertility cases brought to IVF clinics. Male infertility, traditionally viewed as a defect of manhood, can now be perceived as a 'medical condition' treatable in an IVF clinic. Many IVF clinics in the Middle East now advertise ICSI openly as a solution to male infertility. Yet many long-term wives of infertile men are now past the age of providing viable ova for the ICSI procedure. Egg donation or adoption are not options, so infertile Muslim couples with a reproductively elderly wife face the options of remaining permanently without children; remaining together in a polygamous marriage, which is usually not viewed as acceptable by the wives; or divorce, so that the husband can have children with a new and younger marriage partner.

A minority of men are divorcing or taking a second wife as a consequence of the Sunni Islamic restrictions on the use of donor eggs (Inhorn 2007). However, the Shi'ite fatwas allowing egg donation have been a great boon to marital relations in Lebanon, which has a Shi'ite majority. Fertile and infertile men with older wives are streaming into IVF clinics to accept the eggs of donor women. Some of these donors are other IVF patients and some are friends or relatives. Marcia Inhorn (2007) mentions that in at least one clinic some egg donors are non-Muslim, unmarried American women travelling to Lebanon in order to donate their eggs anonymously for a fee to conservative Shi'ite Muslim couples. She also says that some Sunni Muslim patients from Lebanon and other Middle Eastern Muslim countries, such as Egypt and Syria, are surreptitiously crossing transnational borders to rescue their marriages through the use of donor gametes, thereby covertly flouting the dictates of Sunni Muslim orthodoxy. As Inhorn states:

> In short, the arrival of ICSI and donor technologies in the Muslim Middle East has led to a brave new world of reproductive possibilities never imagined when these technologies were first introduced nearly twenty years ago. These technologies have engendered significant medical transnationalism and reproductive tourism; mixing of gametes across ethnic, racial, and religious lines; and the birth of thousands of ICSI and, now, donor babies to devout infertile Muslim couples. (Inhorn 2007:193)

Commercial surrogacy in India

Market dynamics affect how babies and toddlers are brought into families, from assisted reproduction to being sperm or ova, to the purchase of children from poorer countries. Babies can now be received into families through complex arrangements involving lawyers, coordinators, surrogates, 'brokers', donors, sellers, endocrinologists, and without any traditional forms of intimacy (Bratcher Goodwin 2010). Surrogacy is used as a major form of assisted reproduction for westerners travelling abroad to acquire children in China, India, Korea or Ethiopia. Radical feminist scholars have deplored surrogacy as an extreme form of commercialization and technological colonization of women's bodies. They fear that a caste of breeders will arise, comprised of poor, non-white women whose main purpose would be to gestate the embryos of more valuable white women. As an outcome of the economic and patriarchal exploitation of women, the process has been referred to as a kind of prostitution and slavery (Corea 1985; Rothman 1988). However, the impact of assisted reproductive technology on women is multi-layered, with some women becoming agents of control and others being exploited victims (Gupta 2006).

Referring to the case of India, where commercial surrogacy has become a survival strategy and a temporary occupation for some poor rural women, Amrita Pande (2008, 2010) argues that commercial surrogacy is a form of paid labour. Women who work as gestational surrogates in India are involved in a highly stigmatized form of labour. Sex-selective abortions, skewed sex ratios at birth, and high female infanticide and mortality offer persuasive proof of the pervasiveness of son preference in India (see chapter 7). While surrogates are described as angels who help make couples' dreams come true, surrogacy is described as the 'ethics of selling motherhood' and 'renting wombs'. With 30 per cent of the Indians who migrated from India originating from Gujarat, the state has become a key site of medical tourism. Pande (2010) conducted an informative ethnographic study of women's experiences of surrogacy in the small city of Anand in Gujarat. By hiring a surrogate in Anand, clients from all over the world can make significant savings. The cost of a surrogate childbirth in Canada or the USA is between $30,000 and $70,000, whereas in Anand the whole process can cost less than $20,000. Surrogacy in India is not controlled by laws, and fertility clinics such as the one in Anand are directed only by guidelines produced by the Indian Council for Medical Research (ICMR) in 2005. If passed into law, the Assisted Reproductive Technology Regulation Bill and Rules, 2010 will be one of the most accommodating laws on surrogacy globally. In contrast to other countries, the planned law would make surrogacy agreements between the two parties legally enforceable. In the meantime, the clinics that provide ART services may create their own rules.

Among the forty-two surrogates interviewed by Pande, their average family income was near or below the poverty line. For most women who work as surrogates, the $3,000 earned is equivalent to four or five years of their family income. Generally, the education of the women ranged from (self-described) 'illiterate' to high-school level, with the average around the beginning of middle school. Many women had husbands who were unemployed, or employed in informal or temporary labour. As commercial surrogates in India, the women negotiated the anomalies of delivering babies for people from a different class, caste, religion and even race and nation, as well as those associated with surrogacy in general. Women interviewed worked as surrogates for couples from the USA and Europe, as well as emigrant Indian couples who had settled in various nations. Some had been hired by upper-class and middle-class professionals and businesspersons from different states in India.

In most countries, women who work as surrogates are not usually stigmatized, even though gestational surrogacy is questioned on ethical grounds. However, in India, the surrogates face considerable stigma. So almost all the surrogate mothers concealed the knowledge from their communities and parents. They usually hide in the clinic or surrogate hostels in the final stages of pregnancy. Some informed neighbours that the baby was theirs and then said they had miscarried. Most of the surrogates' husbands regarded surrogacy as a familial obligation and not as labour undertaken by the women. However, the media and community often compare surrogates to sex workers. By contrast, in medical discourses surrogacy is viewed as an impersonal contract and surrogates as 'disposable' women (Pande 2010).

One woman who carried a baby for a Mumbai couple said her husband persuaded her to become a surrogate because he needed money to pay the mortgage for his roadside barber's stall. Another who was pregnant for a South Korean couple living in California said she and her husband would use the income to fund their son's heart surgery. Significantly, the surrogate mothers constructed a sense of self-worth by interpreting differences between themselves and others: prostitutes and baby sellers. They defended their husbands' moral worth by comparing them favourably to other men and other husbands. The husbands of women working as surrogates often referred to surrogacy not as a woman's choice or as labour but as a 'team effort' made by the whole family to improve their financial circumstances. They thereby overlooked the essential gendered nature of the work and that the surrogate mothers were doing all the physical and much of the emotional labour. While these explanations oppose the dominant discourse on surrogates as 'immoral sex workers' or 'dirty workers', they also confirm gender hierarchies (Pande 2010).

The process of commercial gestational surrogacy in India emphasizes the disposability of gestational surrogates. The surrogates know that they have no genetic connections with the child and that the baby will be removed from them immediately after delivery. But women working as surrogates resisted these discourses of disposability by emphasizing either their own special attributes or the exceptional bond shared with the hiring couple. The surrogates challenged the anomalous aspects of surrogacy by drawing on cultural symbols to claim a special relationship with the baby (Pande 2008). Despite their narratives of selfless motherhood, Pande emphasizes that the surrogates remain desperately poor Third World women waiting to be saved by their richer, and sometimes whiter, sisters.

Conclusions

Assisted reproduction is generally viewed as a *technological* issue with less consideration of social, political, ethical and legal consequences concerning the creation of new relationships (Culley and Hudson 2009). However, this chapter has explained that NRTs are contentious on several levels. They involve sex, reproduction, nature, parenting, technology, money and religion. Importantly, it demonstrates that NRTs have overturned conventional notions of family ties through use of the technology for *unconventional* family relationships such as gay and lesbian parenting. It also shows that, at the same time, many heterosexual couples have been motivated to use these technologies precisely to try to conform to *conventional* values and religious customs that define traditional family ties. Within both these contradictory aims, new categories of parenthood are being produced which question traditional concepts of biological and social relatedness. The case of the UK Human Fertilization and Embryology Act shows that states attempt to construct, direct and promote normative family structures through government regulation of families created through the use of assisted conception technologies.

The chapter further demonstrates that cultural and religious values and customs can influence couples' engagement with infertility and infertility treatment, as indicated by studies of the cultural values of members of diasporic communities. Women's views are influenced by their religion and gender roles in British South Asian communities (Culley and Hudson 2009). Among couples in western nations, sperm donation is a method used to solve problems of infertility. However, in those societies where fatherhood is strongly defined by biological association, sperm donation is deemed unacceptable. Even though infertility is highly stigmatized among South Asian communities in the UK, donating or receiving gametes is perceived to be far too risky, socially rather than medically.

Similarly, the chapter also explains how the globalization of assisted reproductive technologies and gamete donation generates cultural and religious anxieties in the Middle East. In this region of the world, the recently revised views of male Shi'ite religious leaders towards third-party gamete donation has prompted a transformation in marital relations among infertile Shi'ite Muslim couples, a reconsideration of conventional ideas about biological kinship and parenthood, and the moral tolerance of what were formerly viewed as immoral reproductive acts. Iran, which is governed by a Shi'ite clergy, has been the vanguard of NRTs as a result of new fatwas issued by ostensibly conservative ayatollahs. However, Inhorn (2007) reminds us that most infertile Muslim couples in Iran and elsewhere in the Middle East do not have access to assisted reproductive technologies due the numerous constraints they face. Lack of government investment for these services is understandable given other urgent health problems, including perceived overpopulation. Importantly, since many of the factors leading to infertility among women are both preventable and treatable, investment in prevention is a more desirable use of reproduction technologies (Inhorn 2007).

Recent feminist debates have brought research and debates about infertility and NRTs into the framework of the transnational politics of reproduction. Academic deliberations about surrogacy have mainly concerned moral and ethical issues involving the view that surrogacy leads to subjugation. More recently, debates have extended to examine the impact of surrogacy on the cultural values of motherhood and family, or the motivations that shape surrogacy laws and regulations in western countries such as the UK. The example of surrogacy arrangements and experiences of women in India provides both a macro-social *transnational* dimension and a micro-social *local* dimension that reveal the mechanisms of power, the tensions between women's and men's reproductive agency, and the kinds of cultural and structural inequalities involved in reproductive health.

9 New Directions: Personal Life, Family and Friendship

This final chapter addresses three interrelated themes that comprise threads throughout the book and pose key challenges for sociological studies of family life. The first theme involves the notion of a decline in traditional family values. From the late nineteenth century to the present, sociological theories of family life have echoed versions of this discourse. The decline thesis corresponds with a *family values discourse*, a framework of ideas based on moral anxieties about the fear of a collapse of familial principles and ideals. This discourse, dominant in the USA and UK, is produced by a cluster of prominent public voices including politicians, religious leaders and the media. Although the biological nature of family connections are being challenged and reconfigured by new types of intimacy and belonging, the notion of 'decline' in familial morals has been influential in promoting a nuclear version of the family as the norm (Smart 2007). It has important implications for sociology, given that it has influenced academic debate about family life. Examples of its use in recent political speeches and its social implications are therefore addressed here.

The second set of issues emphasized throughout the book and taken up in this chapter is the call for new sociological concepts and approaches flexible enough to identify and explain the *diversity* in contemporary intimate relationships. New concepts and perspectives, sensitive enough to critique and transcend the notion of 'family decline' are therefore explored here. The term 'personal life' has been developed to emphasize ideas of connectedness about personal relationships, and the fluidity and diversity of contemporary family structures and meanings. The concepts of 'friendship' and 'personal community' are also addressed to demonstrate the way family relations are being rethought and reconfigured. Friendship is used today as a metaphor for changing family relationships. Thus, the terms 'families as friends' and 'friends as family' are increasingly in circulation nowadays to indicate the fluidity and egalitarian possibilities of personal ties. The notion of 'personal communities' has also been developed to explore new ways of approaching family, intimacy and personal life. 'Friendship' and 'personal communities' signal new forms of belonging generated by lesbian, gay, bisexual, transsexual and queer lifestyles which challenge conventional ideas about family and intimate ties.

A third issue addressed in this chapter concerns the need to develop a *global dimension* within sociological approaches to family and intimate life. The intricate and complex web of transnational connections between families and individuals has been highlighted in earlier chapters. A major challenge for family studies in this respect is the use of macro-sociological approaches for an understanding of the relationship between global economies and intimacy. The importance of economic transactions in familial contexts is examined here by addressing the concept of emotional and intimate *exchange* within families and personal life, practised through the obligations of care work and emotion work (Hochschild 1989, 2003b), and the concept of the *purchase of intimacy* (Zelizer 1985, 2005).

The politics of family values

As we have seen in previous chapters, sociological theories about 'the family' from the nineteenth to the twentieth centuries have tended to draw on a white, middle-class ideal as a model against which other family forms were measured. The functionalist approach to the family during the mid twentieth century, outlined in chapter 1, advanced a middle-class 'ideal' and promoted an ethnocentric view of changing family life in which minority-ethnic family patterns were viewed as deviations. Evidence of the continued existence of extended kinship networks among certain classes, minority ethnic groups and in various regions of the world were disregarded by functionalism (Davidoff et al. 1999; Laslett 2005 [1965]). More recently, in the UK and USA, British African Caribbean and African American fatherhood and motherhood have been stigmatized for deviating from the values and practices of white middle-class parenting (Chamberlain 1999; McLoyd et al. 2000). Debates about these social groups have been characterized by stereotypes of 'absent fatherhood' and matriarchal family households, and these views are reflected and perpetuated within family values discourse. The previous chapters explain that these views suggest a lack of understanding of the way race and ethnicity interact with class and culture in parenting practices.

Family values discourse has a long history and continues to flourish today. The public rhetoric of 'family crisis' is not only highly influential in setting the parameters of popular media debate about definitions of the 'proper family', it is also a vote catcher. This rhetoric tends to be drawn on at critical moments of national transition or national crisis such as during times of social disorder and at political elections (Chambers 2001). Notions of family crisis and moral disintegration are expressed in politicians' speeches to evoke the idea that 'the family' either is under siege or is causing a breakdown in the moral fabric of society. Teenage pregnancies, single mothers, absent fathers and bad parenting are regularly highlighted as examples or causes of wider social decline (Stacey 1999; Van Every 1999). Not surprisingly, these public debates have had a strong influence on the formation of social attitudes towards parenting and also on government policy on 'the family' and, in this sense, have an important bearing on sociological studies of family life.

A number of memorable examples over the last half-century illustrate the way 'the family' is used as a political football. For example, in the USA, family values formed a major theme in the presidency of George H.W. Bush. In a televised debate[1] in 1992 he famously called for 'a nation closer to the *Waltons* than the *Simpsons*', presumably to warn about the dangers of dysfunctional American families. In Britain, family values formed the theme in Tony Blair's first major conference speech as Prime Minister in 1997. He identified teenage pregnancies as an example of family breakdown, claiming they undermined the moral fibre of the nation:

> And we cannot say we want a strong and secure society when we ignore its very foundation: family life . . .
>
> Nearly 100,000 *teenage pregnancies* every year. Elderly parents with whom families cannot cope. Children growing up *without role models* they can respect and learn from. More and deeper poverty. More crime. More truancy. More neglect of educational opportunities. And above all, more unhappiness [my emphasis].[2]

The 'lack of role models for children' refers, of course, to the absence of father figures in relation to teenage parenting. President

Bill Clinton echoed this theme in the USA, in 2000, and extended it. He condemned all families that did not conform to two-parent families in a speech on 'Strengthening American Families':

> While the steady reduction in *the number of two-parent families* of the last 40 years has slowed, more than one-third of our children still live in *one-or no-parent families*. There is a high correlation between a childhood spent with *inadequate parental support* and an adulthood spent in poverty or in prison [my emphasis].[3]

George W. Bush also made a number of speeches about the problems of fatherless families and the need for abstinence before marriage, while he was Governor of Texas. His views on family values were crucial to the advancement of his profile leading up to his 2001 US presidency. In a speech about the need to promote responsible fatherhood, Bush declared:

> We're working to mobilize every sector of our society – community leaders and faith-based groups, educators and the media – to increase public awareness of the consequences to children *when fathers are absent*. And we are reaching out to individual men. We want to send this clear message – *every child deserves a father who is committed*, not just legally and financially, but emotionally; an active, loving, *present father*. Every man needs to know that no matter how lofty his job or position, *he will never have a greater duty or more important title than Dad* [my emphasis].[4]

More recently, in the lead-up to his 2009 presidency, Barack Obama took up this family values theme by making a number of speeches about promoting a particular version of 'the family'. He highlighted, again, the problems of single-parent families caused by absent fatherhood:

> Of all the rocks upon which we build our lives, we are reminded today that *family is the most important*. And we are called to recognize and honor *how critical every father is to that foundation. They are teachers and coaches. They are mentors and role models. They are examples of success and the men who constantly push us toward it*. But if we are honest with ourselves, we'll admit that what *too many fathers* also are is *missing* – missing from too many lives and too many homes. They have abandoned their responsibilities, acting like boys instead of men. And *the foundations of our families are weaker* because of it. You and I know how true this is in the African-American community. And the foundations of our community are weaker because of it [my emphasis].[5]

In all these speeches, then, certain kinds of families are identi-fied as 'problem families' and said to threaten the moral fibre of the nation. The key ingredient that validates a moral, stable 'proper family' is the presence of the father. All other family forms are ren-dered suspect or denigrated. Significantly, concerns about the decline of family values underpin a range of government policies in the USA and UK concerning the welfare of families, parenting and children, as mentioned in chapter 3. Government attempts to reduce social welfare costs associated with families headed by women and which have no financial input from fathers are key motives.

More recently still, in August 2011, 'family breakdown' was viewed by the British coalition government as the major cause of the distur-bances on the streets of several English cities. Children and young adults were engaged in rioting, looting and arson which resulted in casualties. The events were initially sparked by a crowd that gathered outside Tottenham police station in London to receive an explana-tion of an unplanned police shooting of a Black man, Mark Duggan, who died. Police initially but mistakenly claimed that Duggan had fired on the police first. Hundreds of young people were arrested and imprisoned after the ensuing riots. A collapse in family morals was judged by the government to be the cause of the social disorder. The notion of a 'broken Britain' was evoked and associated with absent fatherhood, an abandonment of parental responsibility and excessive welfare dependence. Prime Minister David Cameron described the rioting as a 'wake-up call' for the country and promised that the gov-ernment would produce policies that address the causes of 'broken Britain', with the comment:

> Do we have the determination to confront the slow-motion moral collapse that has taken place in parts of our country these past few generations? Irresponsibility. Selfishness. Behaving as if your choices have no conse-quences. Children without fathers. Schools without discipline. Reward without effort. (15 August 2011)[6]

Cameron continued the family breakdown theme in an article in the *Sunday Express* newspaper the following week:

> Above all, a social fightback means instilling in our children and young people the decency, discipline and sense of duty that make good citizens
> . . .
> The first place people learn these values is in the home. That is why I make no apology for talking about the importance of *family and marriage*.

Every government policy must pass what I call the *family test*: does this make *life better for families or worse?* Does this make it easier to bring up well-behaved children or harder? *Family is back at the top of the agenda* [my emphasis].[7]

Underlying explanations about why parents lack the resources to control their children and why young people feel disenfranchised were conspicuously missing from government speeches. The Prime Minister announced that a range of policies would be developed to give support to 120,000 of Britain's 'troubled families' in the wake of the riots.[8] Cameron's 'troubled families' are defined as those with no father: the rioters had no father at home.[9] He went on to state that, in future, he wanted a 'family test' to be applied to all domestic policy.

This range of government responses to the riots contains strong echoes of the discourse of family values half a century earlier in 1960s America, when public figures such as Daniel Patrick Moynihan (1965) embarked on a crusade of criticizing the 'amoral' younger generation (see chapter 1). During that period, the break-up of the 'American family' was blamed on dysfunctional, promiscuous African American families, including single mothers and fatherless families. These examples of political rhetoric about immoral families indicate the current power of this kind of discourse. The 'family values' ideology is, then, highly significant for academic debates about family life. The rhetoric forecloses certain kinds of argument and has fuelled a media-led backlash against certain kinds of families, including single mothers, Black mothers, working mothers, absent fathers, lesbian and gay families and so on (Stacey 1999; Chambers 2001). It encourages ethnocentric views of family and intimate life, with race and gender frequently highlighted as causal factors, through a pattern of blaming single-parent Black families. Through political speeches, public debate and policy, this targeting of non-nuclear families corresponds with an attempt to retrieve a 1950s model of the ideal, white nuclear family.

Family diversity and personal life

The transformations that trouble traditionalists and politicians – including divorce, cohabitation and single parenthood, the demand for more egalitarian relationships by women, and the growth in same-sex unions – are explained by an encroaching individualization and individualistic narcissism, a lack of social responsibility and social cohesion, and an alleged collapse of community. Efforts are now being made in sociology to understand family life in ways that counter this 'decline thesis' and critique the centrality of the conjugal bond, heteronormative frameworks, conventional divisions of labour and ethnocentric notions of family structures.

The growth in a diverse range of intimacies and household arrangements in western and non-western cultures has triggered new sociological conceptualizations of 'family' but has not entailed a discarding of the term 'family' itself. Nevertheless, it is recognized that the conventional use of the term 'family' can lead to reification. It often fails to deal adequately with the ways families are constantly undergoing change in their day-to-day family living. As Morgan (2011:3) states: 'there is no such thing as "The Family"', meaning that we need to avoid the idea of some normative status and shift from the 'cornflake packet' image of the family, given the temptation to measure the divergence of real families from this prevailing image. Thus, while the idea of 'family' is a crucial aspect of the way people reflect upon their personal lives, the difficulty for sociology is that it is instilled with profound symbolic significance, as illustrated by the family values rhetoric above. A number of scholars now challenge the very concept of 'family' for being too hierarchical, patriarchal, homophobic and exclusionary (see, for example, Berlant and Warner 2000; Roseneil and Budgeon 2004; Budgeon 2006).

The trend of familial diversity has been addressed by a number of scholars, including Carol Smart (2007) who uses the concept of *personal life*. The idea of the 'personal' is useful because it avoids the privileging of biological kin or marriage. It confronts the potentially static nature of the term 'family' by including newer family forms and relationships, friendships and reconfigured kinship networks beyond conventionally understood families. The flexibility of this concept allows us, first, to acknowledge that household arrangements are no longer dominated by or confined to the nuclear family form; and, second, to research these diverse arrangements directly. The concept of 'the personal' also has the advantage of not reflecting or being influenced by an idealized model of the white middle-class family. Smart focuses on traditional family ties and wider kinship and yet also on contemporary arrangements such as same-sex partnerships and relationships created through reproductive technologies, LATS (those living apart together) and friendships. Her work comprises a critique of the abstract nature of much recent social theory about families. Smart's preference for the term 'personal' over the term 'individual' also addresses problems associated with the concept of individualization by avoiding the idea of atomized, self-centred individualism.

The concept of 'personal life' corresponds with that of 'family practices' developed by Morgan (2011), discussed in chapter 2. Importantly, both the concepts of 'personal life' and 'family practices' have been generated to acknowledge the inclusion of relationships that are family-like, including friendships. Smart states:

> The 'personal' designates an area of life which impacts closely on people and means much to them, but which does not presume that there is an autonomous individual who makes choices and exercises unfettered agency. This means that the term 'personal life' can invoke the social, indeed it is conceptualised as always already part of the social. (Smart 2007:28)

For Smart, personal life blurs the distinctions between private and public spheres which influence traditional ideas about family life. Families can no longer simply be thought of as distinct households or institutions detached from other locations and structures, especially in post-divorce families, and transnational migrant families where parents are hundreds of miles apart from their children. Smart reminds us that personal life does not have to be thought of as parochial since it is clearly affected by globalization, migration, colonialism and other wider or global processes. It is embedded in and overlaps with public/formal/impersonal life.

Smart raises methodological matters in developing the concept of 'personal life'. 'Personal life' highlights the importance and effectiveness of small-scale, qualitative research, using methods such as ethnography and interviews. Qualitative approaches have the potential to tap into the subtle changes, ambiguities and complexities of personal and family life. These new approaches endorse qualitative studies of personal and family life by emphasizing techniques and traditions of social enquiry characterized by in-depth, open-ended interviews and also including oral histories and life histories, memory work, collective writing projects, the use of visual materials including photographs, and the kind of techniques such as auto/biographical work that allow researchers to be self-reflexive. For example, Jacqui Gabb (2008) has advanced this approach in her book, *Researching*

Intimacy in Families, by developing 'emotional maps' as an innovative research technique to advance the in-depth study of family practices.

Friends and personal communities

Previous chapters have noted that *friends as family* and *family as friends* are terms being used increasingly to describe the fluidity of new kinds of personal relationships that are not necessarily governed by biological ties. Drawing attention to the active agency and reflexive nature of individuals today, Giddens (1992) recognizes 'family' and 'friends' as contexts for the democratization of intimate relationships. The apparently contradictory desires for personal autonomy and the security of family belonging are implied by these terms. Thus, although relationships often remain stratified by gender and age, there is an aspiration for social ties to become more intimate, private and personal. Yet at the same time, given that social ties seem to become more fluctuating and ephemeral, the idea of 'friends as family' seems to match these trends. 'Friends as family' acknowledges a shift in intimate relationships prompted by the increasing changeability, inventiveness and transient nature of social ties in societies characterized by geographical mobility and a rise of people living in single person households. Yet it also implies the growing commitment to and responsibility towards friends. The question is whether *friends* are beginning to overshadow *family* in terms of significance, during late modernity; or whether the concepts of family and friendship are fusing in terms of people's values and actions.

Recent research confirms that more informal and flexible *networks* based on egalitarian relationships are being sought in late modernity and are offering individuals the potential to create new narratives of self. A study by Ray Pahl and Liz Spencer (2001) of the role of friendship in family life suggests that terms such as 'family' and 'friends' are indicative of a commitment to and respect for family relationships. Their findings indicated that 'family' and 'friends' are *converging* categories, with friends becoming more significant in support networks than in the past. Friends, nowadays, often take on certain roles once performed mainly by family. One of the major differences between family and friends is choice (Finch and Mason 1993). Friends are described as *chosen*, while family are perceived as *ascribed*. Pahl and Spencer found that individuals are becoming more selective about which family members they socialize and preserve obligations with.

The question is whether friendship is now overtaking family as a more significant relationship. Outside kinship ties, friends are gradually becoming more important to those who have little contact with their families. This lack of family contact is triggered by the frequency of divorce and separation, the decline of extended kinship ties, the rise of non-heterosexual unions, and the fact that many more people live on their own today. In the UK, for example, the proportion of people who live alone has doubled since the 1970s to 12 per cent as the number of couples with children declines, more people divorce and more delay marriage (Office for National Statistics 2009). This increase crosses all age groups of adults. The prevalent linking of the terms 'family' and 'friends' indicates both the *power* of 'family' as a metaphor for binding friendships as intimate and long-lasting, and the *aspiration* to democratize family relationships. Lynn Jamieson (1998) argues that there has been a historical shift from 'community' to 'intimacy' which persuades us to perceive kin and friendship as analogous relationships 'bound by shared sentiments' (Jamieson 1998:74). However, the growing accent on friendship in family relationships can mask conflict and hierarchies in relationships of kin in the same way that the ideal of the companionate marriage of the early twentieth century concealed gender inequalities (chapter 1).

The term 'friend' is being used increasingly to convey family relationships in which the association is seen as positive and cherished. In the same way, when a friend is perceived as kin, the comparison is also positive and signifies the strength of the bond. However, Pahl and Spencer found that if a friendship is considered a 'duty', then 'family' is a negative term used to describe it as 'family-like'. They found that 'friendship' is being used to endorse cherished family relationships to express the appeal of the bond even though distinctions between family and friends are loosening. Thus, the absence of 'friendship' indicates negative family ties, defined by obligation. Family members are being seen as equivalent to friends if the relationship is perceived as *chosen* rather than a *duty* or if there are strong emotional bonds. Friendship-like ties with family members are now either anticipated as a norm or used as a gauge of the success of family relationships. The value of friendship appears, then, to be escalating alongside a decrease in the importance of extended kin.

A further key concept for the study of the diversity of families and changing intimacies is *personal communities* (Spencer and Pahl 2006).

This describes the range of significant others who are part of our micro-social worlds. Individuals are no longer steeped in extended family or community ties. Rather they tend to draw on a *combination* of 'given' or ascribed (kin) and 'chosen' or elective (friendship) relationships for social support and companionship. Five types of personal community were identified in Spencer and Pahl's study: friend-based; family-based; neighbourhood-based; partner-based; professional-based. The criteria for inclusion were either 'chosen' or 'given' so that, for example, family-based ties and neighbourhood ties were mainly given rather than chosen. However, some individuals have highly permeable personal communities in which friends and family have varied and overlapping roles. Spencer and Pahl (2006:154) conclude that 'it makes little sense to claim that people nowadays have abandoned traditional "families of fate" for "families of choice" based on friends, since the truth, perhaps unsurprisingly, is more complex'.

Among policy-makers, informal yet intense and intimate bonds such as 'personal communities' are now recognized as significant social resources within wider social support networks, as part of *social capital*. Social capital is a form of voluntary association that augments reciprocity and cooperation between individuals for mutual benefit. The concept of social capital is therefore being used in social policy as a value with which to gauge the 'productivity' of community networks, including neighbourhood ties, participation in clubs and voluntary associations (Putnam 2000). The important question posed by Spencer and Pahl's research is whether small circles of micro-social worlds are now the most solid and enduring forms of social capital in contemporary society. If so, does it matter that these personal communities have replaced past forms of social integration that were characterized by traditional community and extended kinship? These questions are yet to be answered by sociologists. Thus, the reconfiguring of traditional ties corresponds with new ideas of the 'self' and 'other', and is generating new ideas about ascribed and chosen relationships (Chambers 2006).

New intimacies

Gay identity politics has advanced debates about ways of subverting the fixed, familial identities conveyed through the family values discourse. The political rhetoric of family values has stigmatized not only single-parent and minority ethnic families but also same-sex couples. Importantly, new patterns of living and new intimacies are moving away from 'family' as a term that encourages prejudice against intimacies that do not conform to the heterosexual and nuclear type of family. The concepts of 'friendship' and 'community' are therefore important metaphors and ways of living used to indicate a move away from conventional heterosexual, nuclear family forms and traditional community associations. The affirmation of sexual identity and distinctive sexual communities in the 1970s was crucial to the gay and lesbian movement and feminism (Weeks 1995) and the rise of queer politics in the 1980s (Weeks et al. 2001).

As a process of new identity formation, 'coming out', as well as taking up residence together, can lead to major changes in personal networks and may entail renegotiations of relationships with existing family and friends. A study of young white college-age women who came out as bisexual or lesbian in the USA, by Ramona Faith Oswald (2000), showed that self-disclosure and questioning of the self and others can lead to a distancing from one's family of origin and increased closeness with friends and peers. She found that, by building a supportive community of like-minded people, individuals could create social networks to help deal with homophobia and heterosexism. While the process of coming out can be distressing for white and western middle-class individuals, for other social groups it can be much more traumatic. For example, among working-class, Muslim and other religious or marginalized groups in which strong kinship ties are dominant, the intersection of sexual and ethnic minority status can lead to distressing circumstances.

A personal community of friends can become a crucial network of support for those engaged in the process of coming out. The process can trigger dramatic changes in relationship arrangements. A study by Andrew Yip (2004) describes how British non-heterosexual Muslims negotiate family and kin in the construction of their identities, and the significant socio-cultural and religious factors involved. Participants talked about the challenges of dealing with the strict religious censure of homosexuality based on various Islamic written sources, and the pervasive cultural censure of homosexuality as a 'western disease'. The expectation of marriage as a cultural and religious obligation, the respect for parents, and the maintenance of family honour (*izzat*), especially in close-knit kinship networks, were all factors that shaped participants' responses and experiences.

Secrecy, silence and discretion had to be observed in balancing socio-religious obligations against the aspiration to express sexuality. In these kinds of circumstances, non-kin friendships can form crucial support networks.

Friendship plays a significant role in 'families of choice' (Weeks et al. 2001), but the idea that friendship may act as a surrogate family has not been assumed in all gay and lesbian unions. Thus, while Weeks et al. (2001) embrace the notion of 'family' as well as 'friendship' to describe the emergent nature of GLBT intimacies (see chapter 2), others, such as Berlant and Warner (2000), view the term 'families of choice' as highly conservative and integrationist. While friendship provides a vital source of support for those who have been rejected by relatives after having taken on a non-heterosexual identity, many object to the association of the term 'friendship' with the concept of 'family' to describe same-sex relationships. For many, 'family' evokes hierarchy, bigotry and constraint. Since several self-identified non-heterosexual people have become reliant on chosen relationships with friends after being shunned by their families of origin, it is not surprising that, as Weeks et al. (2001:11) state, 'people slide easily between viewing the family as a site of hostility, and as something they can invent'. They point out that 'Friends are *like* family; or they *are* family. The family is something external to you, or something you do' (Weeks et al. 2001:11). The power of family values rhetoric in hijacking a particular version of 'family' indicates the difficulties entailed for those who wish to use the same language to contest the ideological norms that attempt to regulate social and personal relationships (Weeks et al. 2001).

The more fluid nature of the term 'friendship', compared to that of 'family', foregrounds the diversity of relationships in queer cultures. The concept seems to hold the promise of blurring the boundaries between the sexual and the non-sexual. The term 'non-standard intimacies' is used to symbolize a break away from the hierarchical relationships often implied by the term 'family'(Budgeon and Roseneil 2002). Berlant and Warner (2000) emphasize the counter-normative nature and radical potential of many such relationships. Non-heterosexual politics has stressed the radical democratization of personal relationships that Giddens (1992) refers to as a 'pure relationship' (chapter 2). However, although Giddens emphasized the freedom to choose new living arrangements outside the traditional family, he did not address the fact that commitment and care are often as central to new intimacies and living arrangements as the democratizing impulse (Roseneil and Budgeon 2004).

A problem associated with the search for new concepts to analyse and understand changes in personal and family life is that power relations and inequalities of gender, race, age and ethnic identity can be neglected while highlighting the strengths of family and personal commitments and reciprocities. There is nothing intrinsically ethnocentric about the concepts of 'personal life', 'family practices', 'personal communities', 'friends as family' or 'families of choice'. However, given that these terms foreground the agency of personhood in contemporary western societies, we need to ensure that they are not used in such a way as to be narrowly relevant to white, middle-class ideas of identity experimentation and agency. Experimentation with personal identity, embedded in the idea of the 'self as project', can sometimes appear to exist outside class, gender and racial inequalities. As mentioned in chapter 2, research on working-class lesbian couples with children demonstrates the class-related difficulties of overcoming the stigma of being lesbian parents (Taylor 2007).

Global and economic dimensions of intimacy and family

A wider set of issues concerning the 'self as project' are opened up by extending our focus to a global stage. Debates about changes in personal and family life, obligation of care and ageing populations are linked to changing ideas about the relationship between the self and society. Across the globe, we find that traditional and late modern notions of the self are in tension with one another. These tensions can have far-reaching consequences for changing family dynamics and personal relations when negotiated across great distances (Durham 2007). Traditional concepts of 'self', based on *family duties* and *intergenerational reciprocity*, collide with contemporary western values of 'the individual' associated with *liberal individualism* and *self-autonomy*, even though studies of western intimacies and kin ties demonstrate commitment and reciprocity. Nevertheless, the tensions arising from these divergent concepts of the self correspond with differing approaches to *family-based* welfare and *public* welfare which have shaped support systems for older populations in richer and poorer nations (see Cole and Durham 2007). Western values of individual autonomy are being fostered by neoliberal economic and state policies in Third World contexts through NGOs, and being promoted by international organizations such as the International Monetary Fund and the World Bank (Durham 2007:103).

A further challenge is that global approaches to the study of family life seem to be located at the opposite end of the spectrum from those focused on individual self-autonomy. A western emphasis on individualism can make it difficult for western observers to appreciate the important way in which *intimacies* are shaped through family-based *economic transactions* in other parts of the globe. The integration of economic transactions with intimate practices has been addressed in chapter 6 in relation to commercial marriage transactions and care migration, and in chapter 8 with regard to the purchase of babies through commercial surrogacy and other reproductive technologies. These sections demonstrate that across the world, *affective* payments – which centrally involve emotions and intimacies – are considered acceptable forms of social transaction in courtship and marriage, in caring relationships, in adoption and assisted reproduction.

However, global considerations of family life tend to involve wider, *macro-sociological* perspectives with attention focused on public spheres, whereas approaches that address the diversity of family and personal life in the West tend to rely on *micro-sociological*, often qualitative methods and a focus on private, domestic spheres. Economic transactions and intimate personal relations are inextricably interconnected through caring economies and affective work. Thus, global approaches to family studies are now also being advanced in order to address the relationship between the 'public' worlds of politics and work and the 'private' worlds of intimacy/family (Nelson 1998; Hochschild 2003b; Zelizer 2005). In this final section of the volume, the structuring of *emotion exchanges* in personal and family life is addressed as an example of the way these domains are interconnected and brought together through the study of intimate life.

As chapter 6 demonstrates, individuals and families are being pressured to adapt to the needs of global capital. As such, they often find it more difficult to fulfil duties of care to their ageing kin, across great distances. Research on transnational kinship and communities demonstrates how families maintain support across geographical distances (Baldassar 2007). However, there are significant gaps in social policy, both in countries with high numbers of emigrants and in those with high numbers of immigrants. Elderly relatives left behind are often in need of support from states that do not traditionally have welfare provision for the elderly. Those individuals and families moving to new countries to find employment may either be vulnerable to welfare needs as they move to retirement age, or have to consider bringing over their parents in order to look after them in old age, or travelling back to their country of origin to retire. Thus, sociological studies of personal and family life require the inclusion of a transnational framework to take account of the major pressures of care provision placed on migrant individuals, transnational families and diasporic communities. Yet there is also a need for small-scale, qualitative research on transnational care to understand how families cope, and the effects on children and the elderly of wider global patterns of change.

Examples of the kind of work that crosses local/global boundaries and macro-/micro-social perspectives include research by Arlie Hochschild and Viviana Zelizer. The terms *emotion work* and the *care deficit* are used by Hochschild (1989, 2003b) to address the gendered nature of issues that affect women in their roles in families (chapter 6). More recently, she has argued that family relations are structured by the gendering of *exchanges of emotion* (Hochschild 2003b). This corresponds with feminist research that explains how women uphold and sustain families and households through their domestic labour, thereby supporting relationships between fathers and children (Delphy and Leonard 1992; Seery and Crowley 2000). Hochschild (2003b) highlights the intricate connections between public and private worlds by combining the emotional and the economic in her analysis of an affective *economy of gratitude*. Individuals engage in 'gift' emotion work to others as an affective exchange that transcends necessity in an 'economy of gratitude'. She emphasizes that an economy of gratitude is an almost sacred dimension of an intimate bond which is essential to the organization of personal and family life. In heterosexual familial contexts, the kind of mutual exchange involved is gender-bound, determined by gendered roles and expectations. For example, if the father provides childcare it is often interpreted as a gift to the mother, but not so if the mother provides it since it is expected of her as her duty.

Women also regularly perform the emotional work in families by doing the work of 'keeping in touch' with relatives and sustaining the relationship between fathers and their children (Leonardo 1987). As Gabb (2008:91) states: 'The activities that women routinely do, such as feeding the family, not only serve a pragmatic purpose, but also perform a symbolic function, with mothers literally constructing a sense of family through their everyday family role.' The way women uphold relationships between fathers and children is demonstrated more dramatically by research outlined in chapter 7 on fertility and population policies, and chapter 8 on reproductive technologies. Customs such as son preference and population policies regulate women's bodily encounters and well-being in the context of fertility through abortions, IVF and other reproductive technologies. These practices and forms of regulation of women's bodies support the demands and expectations of husbands and their kin in the creation of desired family forms to duplicate or represent 'biological' ties.

Like Hochschild, Zelizer (2005) focuses on the financial value of relational care and undertakes an economic analysis of the role of emotion/intimacy or 'affect' in economic exchanges. She argues that the expansion of world markets corresponds with an intrusion of commercial social relations in every area of our personal lives. Zelizer (2005) argues that, contrary to popular western myths, the idea that there is a moral separation between *economy* and *intimacy* does not follow where intimacy and families are concerned. Examples in earlier chapters that bear this out include the payment for surrogacy, egg donations, arranged marriages, mail-order brides and the purchase of care by wealthy families across the world. These are profoundly intimate social transactions which are nevertheless regulated and framed as monetary transactions. As Zelizer (2005:28) emphasizes, intimate relations are configured by financial transfers that are then integrated into global webs of mutual obligations. She refers to the *purchase of intimacy* to draw attention to economic exchanges of intimate care and how these combine with meanings given to practices of care and affect. Indeed, the financial and emotional value placed on care by western societies is demonstrated by the processes through which they are regulated. They are regulated in the context of divorce through social policy and contested through law. The 'purchase of intimacy' approach contributes to an understanding of the ways the *public* and *private* coalesce. Thus, analyses of intimate practices and care can help us to recognize the complex intersections between private, familial, personal and intimate spheres of life and public, global and economic spheres of society.

Notes

2 Individualization, Intimacy and Family Life

1 Information about CAVA: Care, Values and the Future of Welfare is available at www.leeds.ac.uk/cava/aboutcava/aboutcava.htm (accessed 19 August 2011).

4 The Changing Nature of Childhoood

1 United Nations Convention on the Rights of the Child, available at www2. ohchr.org/english/law/pdf/crc.pdf (accessed 22 February 2011).
2 See 'Global initiative to end all corporal punishment of children', available at www.endcorporalpunishment.org/pages/progress/prohib_states. html (accessed 21 August 2011).

5 Families and Ageing Societies

1 Indians emigrated to the USA in response to the 1965 US Immigration and Naturalization Act which increased immigration opportunities for people from Asia.
2 'Patrilineal' refers to a system in which a person belongs to their father's lineage rather than their mother's lineage. It generally entails the inheritance of property, names or titles through the male line. 'Matriarchal' refers to a system in which a person belongs through the mother-line.
3 'Filial': the relationship of the offspring to the parent.

6 Globalization, Migration and Intimate Relations

1 Serial migration, also known as 'chain migration', is defined as a movement in which prospective migrants hear about opportunities and are supplied with transportation, preliminary accommodation and employment which are organized through their relationships with previous migrants.

2 'Endogamous' refers to the social practice of marrying another member of the same clan, people or other kinship group.

7 Families, Fertility and Populations

1 National Policy for the Empowerment Of Women available at wcd.nic.in/empwomen.htm (accessed 11 December 2011).

8 Families and New Reproductive Technologies

1 Gametes are the reproductive cells of men and women: the male sperm and the female eggs (or ova).
2 A fatwa is an Islamic religious ruling issued by a recognized religious authority.

9 New Directions: Personal Life, Family and Friendship

1 National Religious Broadcasters, January 1992.
2 Press release of 'Text of speech by Right Honourable Tony Blair at Labour Party Annual Conference, Brighton, October 1997'. Available at www.prnewswire.co.uk/cgi/news/release?id=47983 (accessed 15 August 2011).
3 The Hyde Park Declaration oo–DLC4 on 1 August 2000; available at www.ontheissues.org/Notebook/Note_00–DLC4.htm (accessed 15 August 2011).
4 Press Release, 'National summit on fatherhood', 2 June 2000, available at www.presidency.ucsb.edu/ws/index.php?pid=45956#axzz1V60KElPi (accessed 15 August 2011).
5 Chicago Church speech, 15 June 2008, in *Obama* (2008:234–5).
6 Allegra Stratton, 'David Cameron on riots: broken society is top of my political agenda', 15 August 2011, including video of Cameron's speech, available at www.guardian.co.uk/uk/2011/aug/15/david-cameron-riots-broken-society (accessed 11 December 2011).
7 David Cameron, 'Human rights in my sights', *Sunday Express*, 21 August 2011, available at www.express.co.uk/posts/view/266219/David-Cameron-Human-rights-in-my-sights (accessed 11 December 2011).
8 See 'England riots: Cameron to boost troubled families plan', *BBC News*, 15 August 2011, available at www.bbc.co.uk/news/uk-politics-14527540 (accessed 11 December 2011).
9 Ibid.

Bibliography

Abraham, M. (2008) Domestic violence and the Indian diaspora in the United States. In R. Palriwala and P. Uberoi (eds.) *Marriage, Migration and Gender*. New Delhi: Sage, pp. 303–25.

ActionAid (2008) *Disappearing Daughters: India Sex Selection Crisis Worsening*. Available online at www.actionaid.org.uk/doc_lib/disappearing_daughters_0608.pdf (accessed 14 April 2011).

Adams, P. C. and Ghose, R. (2003) India.com: the construction of a space between. *Progress in Human Geography* **27** (4), 414–37.

Adams, R. and Blieszner, R. (eds.) (1989) *Older Adult Friendship: Structure and Process*. Newbury Park: Sage.

Agarwal, B. (1994) *A Field of One's Own: Gender and Land Rights in South Asia*. Cambridge: Cambridge University Press.

Alcock, P. (1997) *Understanding Poverty*. Basingstoke: Macmillan.

Allan, G. (1996) *Kinship and Friendship in Modern Britain*. Oxford: Oxford University Press.

Allan, G. and Crow, G. (2001) *Families, Households and Society*. London: Palgrave.

Allgar, V., Atkin, K., Din, I. and Mcnesh, D. (2003) *Ethnicity and Parenting: A Review of Literature and Investigation Based on Secondary Analysis*. York: Joseph Rowntree Foundation.

Almack, K. (2008) Display work: lesbian parent couples and their families of origin negotiating new kin relationships. *Sociology* **42**, 1183–99.

Almack, K., Seymour, J. and Bellamy, G. (2010) Exploring the impact of sexual orientation on experiences and concerns about end of life care and on bereavement for lesbian, gay and bisexual older people. *Sociology* **44**, 908–92.

Amato, P. R. and DeBoer, D. D. (2001) The transmission of marital instability across generations: relationship skills or commitment to marriage? *Journal of Marriage and the Family* **63**, 1038–51.

Amato, P. R. and Keith, B. (1991) Parental divorce and the well-being of children: a meta-analysis. *Psychological Bulletin* **110**, 26–46.

Anagnost, A. (2008) Imagining global futures in China: the child as a sign of value. In J. Cole and D. Durham (eds.) *Figuring the Future: Globalization and the Temporalities of Children and Youth*. Santa Fe, NM: School for Advanced Research Press, pp. 49–73.

Arai, L. (2003) Low expectations, sexual attitudes and knowledge: explaining teenage pregnancy and fertility in English communities. Insights from qualitative research. *Sociological Review* 5, 199–217.

Arber, S. and Attias-Donfut, C. (eds.) (1999) *The Myth of Generational Conflict: The Family and State in Ageing Societies*. London: Routledge.

Arber, S. and Ginn, J. (1991) *Gender and Later Life: A Sociological Analysis of Resources and Constraints*. London: Sage.

Archer, L. (2003) *'Race', Masculinity and Schooling: Muslim Boys and Education*. Buckingham: Open University Press.

Ariès, P. (1962) *Centuries of Childhood: A Social History of Family Life*. London: Cape.

Arnold, E. (2004) Broken attachments of women from the West Indies separated from mothers in early childhood. Unpublished Ph.D. thesis, University College, London University.

Arnold, F., Choe, M. K. and Roy, T. K. (1998) Son preference, the family-building process and child mortality in India. *Population Studies* 52, 301–15.

Aschbrenner, J. (1978) Continuities and variations in Black family structures. In D. B. Shimkin, E. M. Shimkin and D. A. Frate (eds.) *The Extended Family in Black Societies*. The Hague: Mouton, pp. 181–200.

Atkinson, K., Oerton, S. and Burns, D. (1998) Happy families? Single mothers, the press and the politicians. *Capital and Class* 64, 1–11.

Bailey, J. (2003) *Unquiet Lives: Marriage and Marriage Breakdown in England, 1660–1800*. Cambridge: Cambridge University Press.

Baldassar, L. (2007) Transnational families and aged care: the mobility of care and the migrancy of ageing. *Journal of Ethnic and Migration Studies* 33, 275–97.

Ball, S. J., Bowe, R. and Gewirtz, S. (1996) School choice, social class and distinction: the realization of social advantage in education. *Journal of Education Policy* 11, 89–112.

Barlow, A., Duncan, S., James, G. and Park, A. (2005) *Cohabitation, Marriage and the Law: Social Change and Legal Reform in the 21st Century*. Oxford: Hart.

Barn, R. with Ladino, C. and Rogers, B. (2006) *Parenting in Multi-racial Britain*. The Parenting in Practice series. London: National Children's Bureau.

Barrett, M. (1980) *Women's Oppression Today*. London: Verso.

Barrett, M. and McIntosh, M. (1982) *The Anti-Social Family*. London: Verso.

Bauer, E. and Thompson, P. (2006) *Jamaican Hands Across the Atlantic*. Kingston, Jamaica: Ian Randle Publishers.

Bauman, Z. (2003) *Liquid Love: On the Frailty of Human Bonds*. Cambridge: Polity Press.

Beattie, J. H. M. (1964) Kinship and social anthropology. *Man* **64** (130), 101–3.

Beck-Gernsheim, E. (2002) *Reinventing the Family: In Search of New Lifestyles*. Cambridge: Polity Press.

Beck, U. (1992) *Risk Society: Towards a New Modernity*. London: Sage.

Beck, U. (1994) The reinvention of politics: towards a theory of reflexive modernisation. In U. Beck and S. Lash, *Reflexive Modernisation: Politics, Tradition and Aesthetics in the Modern Social Order*. Cambridge: Polity Press, pp.1–55.

Beck, U. and Beck-Gernsheim, E. (1995) *The Normal Chaos of Love*. Cambridge: Polity Press.

Beck, U. and Beck-Gernsheim, E. (2002) *Individualization: Institutionalized Individualism and its Social and Political Consequences*. London: Sage.

Beeson, D. (1975) Women in studies of ageing: a critique and suggestion. *Social Problems*, 52–9.

Bell, C. (1968) *Middle Class Families*. London: Routledge & Kegan Paul.

Bengtson, V. L., Biblarz, T. J. and Roberts, R. E. L. (2002) *How Families Still Matter: A Longitudinal Study of Youth in Two Generations*. Cambridge: Cambridge University Press.

Bentley, G. R. and Mascie-Taylor, N. (eds.) (2000) *Infertility in the Modern World: Present and Future Prospects*. Cambridge: Cambridge University Press.

Berlant, L. and Warner, M. (2000) Sex in public. In L. Berlant (ed.) *Intimacy*. Chicago: University of Chicago Press, pp. 311–30.

Bernard, J. (1974) *The Future of Motherhood*. New York: Dial Press.

Bharadwaj, A. (2003) Why adoption is not an option in India: the visibility of infertility, the secrecy of donor insemination, and other cultural complexities. *Social Science and Medicine* **56**, 1867–80.

Biao, X. (2008) Gender, dowry and the migration system of Indian information technology professionals. In R. Palriwala and P. Uberoi (eds.) *Marriage, Migration and Gender*. New Delhi: Sage, pp. 235–60.

Biblarz, T. J and Savci, E. (2010) Lesbian, gay, bisexual, and transgender families. *Journal of Marriage and Family* **72**, 480–97.

Billingsley, A. (1968) *Black Families in White America*. Englewood Cliffs, NJ: Prentice Hall.

Blanchet, T. (2008) Bangladeshi girls sold as wives in North India. In R. Palriwala and P. Uberoi (eds.) *Marriage, Migration and Gender*. New Delhi: Sage, pp. 152–79.

Boal, F. (ed.) (2000) *Ethnicity and Housing*. Aldershot: Ashgate.

Bonvalet, C. and Ogg, J. (eds.) (2007) *Measuring Family Support in Europe*. London: Southern Universities Press.

Borooah, V. and Iyer, S. (2004) *Religion and Fertility in India: The Role of Son Preference and Daughter Aversion*. Cambridge: Department of Applied Economics, University of Cambridge.

Bourdieu, P. (1977) *Reproduction in Education, Society and Culture*. London: Sage.

Bourdieu, P. (1983) The forms of capital. In J. G. Richardson (ed.) *Handbook of Theory and Research for the Sociology of Education*. New York: Greenwood Press, pp. 241–58.

Bourdieu, P. (1986) *Distinction: A Social Critique of the Judgement of Taste*. London: Routledge.

Bourdieu, P. (2004) Forms of capital. In S. Ball (ed.) *The Routledge Falmer Reader in Sociology of Education*. London: Routledge Falmer.

Bovill, M. and Livingstone, S. (2001) Bedroom culture and the privatization of media use. In S. Livingstone and M.Bovill (eds.) *Children and their Changing Media Environment: A European Comparative Study*. Mahwah, NJ: Lawrence Erlbaum Associates, pp. 179–200.

Bowlby, J. (1953) *Child Care and the Growth of Love*. London: Penguin.

Brandth, B. and Kvande, E. (2003) *Fleksible fedre: maskulinitet, arbeid, velferdsstat (Flexible Fathers: Masculinity, Work, Welfare State)*. Oslo: Universitetsforlaget.

Branigan, T. (2008) Days of the one-child rule could be numbered as Beijing considers change. *The Guardian*, 29 February 2008.

Brannen, J. and Nilsen, A. (2005) Individualisation, choice and structure: a discussion of current trends in sociological analysis. *Sociological Review* **53**, 412–28.

Brannen, J. and Nilsen, A. (2006) From fatherhood to fathering: transmission and change among British fathers in four-generation families. *Journal of Sociology* **40** (2), 335–52.

Brannen, J. and O'Brien, M. (eds.) (1996) *Children in Families: Research and Policy*. London: Falmer Press.

Brannen, J., Dodd, K., Oakley, A. and Storey, P. (1994) *Young People, Health and Family Life*. Buckingham: Open University Press.

Bratcher Goodwin, M. (2010) *Baby Markets: Money and the New Politics of Creating Families*. Cambridge: Cambridge University Press.

Brookdale Center on Aging (1999) *Assistive Housing for Elderly Gays and Lesbians in New York City*. New York: Brookdale Center on Aging and Senior Action in a Gay Environment (Sage).

Brotman S., Ryan, B. and Cormier, R. (2003) The health and social services needs of gay and lesbian elders and their families in Canada. *The Gerontologist* **43**, 192–202.

Buckingham, D. (2007). *Beyond Technology: Children's Learning in the Age of Digital Media*. Cambridge: Polity Press.

Budgeon, S. (2006) Friendship and formations of sociality in late modernity:

the challenge of 'post-traditional intimacy'. *Sociological Research Online*, 11 (3). Available online at www.socresonline.org.uk/11/3/budgeon.html (accessed 11 December 2011).

Budgeon, S. and Roseneil, S. (2002) Cultures of intimacy and care beyond 'The Family': friendship and sexual/love relationships in the twenty-first century. Paper presented at the International Sociological Association World Congress of Sociology, Brisbane, July 2002. Available online at www.leeds.ac.uk/cava/papers/culturesofintimacy.htm (accessed 11 December 2011).

Bulmer, M. and Solomos, J. (eds.) (1999) *Racism*. Oxford: Oxford University Press.

Burgess, E. (1973) *On Community, Family and Delinquency*. Chicago: University of Chicago Press.

Burgess, E. and Locke, H. J. (1945) *The Family: From Institution to Companionship*. New York: American Book Company.

Burghes, L. (1994) *Lone Parenthood and Family Disruption*. London: Family Policy Studies Centre.

Butler, J. (1999 [1990]) *Gender Trouble: Feminism and the Subversion of Identity*. New York: Routledge.

Cabinet Office [now at Department for Education] (2008) *Families in Britain: an evidence paper*. Available online at www.education.gov.uk/publications/standard/publicationdetail/page1/dcsf-01077–2008 (accessed 28 April 2011).

Cahill, S., South, K. and Spade, J. (2000) *Outing Age: Public Policy Issues Affecting Gay, Lesbian, Bisexual and Transgendered Elders*. Washington, DC: National Gay and Lesbian Task Force Policy Unit.

Carrington, C. (1999) *No Place Like Home: Relationships and Family Life Among Lesbians and Gay Men*. Chicago and London: University of Chicago Press.

Casper, L. and Bianchi, S. (2002) *Continuity and Change in the American Family*. Thousand Oaks, CA: Sage.

Castles, S. and Miller, M. (1998) *The Age of Migration: International Population Movements in the Modern World*. London: Macmillan.

Chadwick, A. and Heffernan, R. (2003) *The New Labour Reader*. Cambridge: Polity Press.

Chamberlain, M. (1995) Family narratives and migration dynamics. *New West Indies Guide / Nieue West Indische Gids* **69**, 253–75.

Chamberlain, M. (1999) Brothers and sisters, uncles and aunts: a lateral perspective on Caribbean families. In E. Silva and C. Smart (eds.) *The New Family?* London: Sage, pp. 129–42.

Chamberlain, M. (2001) Migration, the Caribbean and the family. In H. Goulbourne and M. Chamberlain (eds.) *Caribbean Families in the TransAtlantic World*. London: Macmillan, pp. 32–47.

Chamberlain, M. (2003) Rethinking Caribbean families: extending the links. *Community, Work and Family* **6**, 63–76.

Chambers, D. (2001) *Representing the Family*. London: Sage.

Chambers, D. (2006) *New Social Ties: Contemporary Connections in a Fragmented Society*. London: Palgrave Macmillan.

Chambers, D. (2011) 'Wii play as family': the rise in family-centred video gaming. *Leisure Studies*, 4 July 2011, 1–14. Available online at www.tandfonline.com/doi/abs/10.1080/02614367.2011.568065.

Chambers, D., Steiner, L. and Fleming, C. (2004a) *Women and Journalism*. London: Routledge.

Chambers, D., Tincknell, E. and Van Loon, J. (2004b) Peer regulation of teenage sexual identities. *Gender and Education*, **16** (3), 397–415.

Chambers, P., Allan, G., Phillipson, C. and Ray, M. (2009) *Family Practices in Later Life*. Bristol: Policy Press.

Chapman, T. (2004) *Gender and Domestic Life: Changing Practices in Families and Households* London: Palgrave Macmillan.

Charsley, K. (2008) Vulnerable brides and transnational *Ghar Damads*: gender, risk and 'adjustment' among Pakistani marriage migrants to Britain. In R. Palriwala and P. Uberoi (eds.) *Marriage, Migration and Gender*. New Delhi: Sage, pp. 261–85.

Cheale, D. (1999) The one and the many: modernity and postmodernity. In G. Allan (ed.) *The Sociology of the Family: A Reader*. Oxford: Basil Blackwell.

Cheale, D. (2002) *Sociology of Family Life*. London: Palgrave.

Cheong, P. H. (2008) The young and techless? Investigating internet use and problem-solving behaviours of young adults in Singapore. *New Media and Society* **10**, 771–91.

Child Trends (2010) Child trends indicators, from *Child Trends DataBank*. http://childtrendsdatabank.org.

ChildWise (2009) *The Monitor Report 2008–9: Children's Media Use and Purchasing*. Norwich: ChildWise.

Chin, E. (2001) *Purchasing Power: Black Kids and American Consumer Culture*. Minneapolis: University of Minnesota Press.

Chodorow, N. (1978) *The Reproduction of Mothering: Psychoanalysis and the Sociology of Gender*. Berkeley, CA: University of California Press.

Chou, R. J. A. (2010) Willingness to live in eldercare institutions among older adults in urban and rural China: a nationwide study. *Ageing & Society* **30**, 583–608.

Cockett, M. and Tripp, J. (1994) *The Exeter Family Study: Family Breakdown and its Impact on Children*. Exeter: University of Exeter Press.

Cole, J. (2001) *Loving Yourself Loving Another: The Importance of Self-esteem for Successful Relationships*. London: Vermilion.

Cole, J. and Durham, D. (2007) *Generations and Globalisation: Youth, Age and*

Family in the New World Economy. Bloomington and Indianapolis: Indiana University Press.

Cole, J. W. and Nydon, J. A. (1990) Class, gender and fertility: contradictions of social life in contemporary Romania. *East European Quarterly* **23**, 469–76.

Collier, R. (1999) Men, heterosexuality and the changing family: (re)constructing fatherhood in law and social policy. In G. Jagger and C. Wright (eds.) *Changing Family Values*. London: Routledge, pp. 38–58.

Collier, R. (2005) Fathers 4 justice, law and the new politics of fatherhood. *Child and Family Law Quarterly* **17**, 1–29.

Collier, R. and Sheldon, S. (2008) *Fragmenting Fatherhood: A Socio-legal Study*. Oxford and Portland, Oregon: Hart Publishing.

Constable, N. (2003). *Romance on a Global Stage: Pen Pals, Virtual Ethnography, and 'Mail-Order' Marriages*. Berkeley, CA: University of California Press.

Corea, G. (1985) *The Mother Machine: Reproductive Technologies from Artificial Insemination to Artificial Wombs*. New York: Harper and Row.

Corsaro, W. A. (1997) *The Sociology of Childhood*. Thousand Oaks, CA: Pine Forge Press.

Coulthard, M. and Walker, A. (2002) *People's Perceptions of Their Neighbourhoods and Community Involvement: Results from the Social Capital Module of the General Household Survey, 2000*. London: The Stationery Office.

Coward, R. (1983) *Patriarchal Precedents: Sexuality and Social Relations*. London: Routledge & Kegan Paul.

Craig, L. (2007) *Contemporary Motherhood: The Impact of Children on Adult Time*. Aldershot: Ashgate Publishing.

Critcher, C. (2008) Making waves: historical aspects of public debates about children and mass media. In K. Drotner and S. Livingstone (eds.) *The International Handbook of Children, Media and Culture*. London: Sage, pp. 91–104.

Croll, E. (2000) *Endangered Daughter: Discrimination and Development in Asia*. London: Routledge.

Crow, G. (2002) Families, moralities, rationalities and social change. In A. Carling, S. Duncan and R. Edwards (eds.) *Analysing Families*. London: Routledge, pp. 285–97.

Crow, G. and Allan, G. (1994) *Community Life: An Introduction to Local Social Relationships*. Hemel Hempstead: Harvester Wheatsheaf.

Crozier, G. (1996) Empowering the powerful: a discussion of the interrelation of government policies and consumerism with social class factors and the impact of this upon parent interventions in their children's schooling. *British Journal of Sociology of Education* **18**, 87–200.

Culley, L. and Hudson, N. (2006) Diverse bodies and disrupted reproduction: infertility and minority ethnic communities in the UK. *International*

Journal of Diversity in Organisations, Communities and Nations **5** (2), 117–26.

Culley, L. and Hudson, N. (2009) Constructing relatedness: ethnicity, gender and third party assisted conception in the UK. *Current Sociology* **57**, 249–67.

Culley, L., Hudson, N., Rapport, F., Katbamna, S. and Johnson, M. (2007) 'I know about one treatment where they keep the egg somewhere': British South Asian community understandings of infertility and its treatment. *Diversity in Health and Social Care* **4** (2): 113–21.

Cunningham, H. (1995) *Children and Childhood in Western Society since 1500*. Harlow: Longman.

Daatland, S. O. and Herlofson, K. (2003) 'Lost solidarity' or 'changed solidarity': a comparative European view of normative family solidarity. *Ageing and Society* **23**, 537–61.

Dallos, R. and McLaughlin, E. (eds.) (1993) *Social Problems and the Family*. Newbury Park: Sage.

Dalton, S. and Bielby, D. (2000) 'That's our kind of constellation': lesbian mothers negotiate institutionalized understandings of gender within the family. *Gender and Society* **14** (February), 36–61.

Davidoff L., Doolittle, M., Fink, J. and Hoden, K. (1999) *The Family Story: Blood, Contract and Intimacy, 1830–1960*. London: Longman.

Davin, D. (2008) Marriage migration in China: the enlargement of marriage markets in the era of market reforms. In R. Palriwala and P. Uberoi (eds.) *Marriage, Migration and Gender*. New Delhi: Sage, pp. 63–77.

Delphy, C. (1977) Towards a materialist feminism? *Feminist Review* 1, 95–105.

Delphy, C. and Leonard, D. (1992) *Familiar Exploitation*. Cambridge: Polity Press.

Del Rosario, T. (2008) Bridal diaspora: migration and marriage among Filipino women. In R. Palriwala and P. Uberoi (eds.) *Marriage, Migration and Gender*. New Delhi: Sage, pp. 98–124.

Demos, D. H. and Cox, M. J. (2000) Families with young children: a review of research in the 1990s. *Journal of Marriage and the Family* **62**, 876–95.

Dench, G. (1996) *The Place of Men in Changing Family Attitudes*. London: Institute of Community Studies.

Dench, G. and Ogg, J. (2002) *Grandparenting in Britain*. London: Institute of Community Studies.

Dennis, N., Henriques, F. and Slaughter, C. (1956) *Coal is Our Life: An Analysis of a Yorkshire Mining Community*. London: Tavistock.

Department of Education and Science (1985) *The Swann Report, 'Education for All', Report of the Committee of Enquiry into the Education of Children from Ethnic Minority Groups*. London: HMSO. Available online at: www.educationengland.org.uk/documents/swann/ (accessed 1 August 2011).

Department of Health (2008) *End of Life Care Strategy: Promoting High Quality Care for all Adults at the End of Life.* London: Department of Health.

Department of Trade and Industry (DTI) (2003) *Equality and Diversity: Age Matters.* London: Department of Trade and Industry.

Dermott, E. (2003) The 'intimate father': defining paternal involvement. *Sociological Research Online* 8 (4). Available online at www.socresonline. org.uk/8/4/dermott.html (accessed February 2008).

Dermott, E. (2008) *Intimate Fatherhood.* London: Routledge.

Devine, F. (1992) *Affluent Workers Revisited: Privatism and the Working Class.* Edinburgh: Edinburgh University Press.

De Vries, B. (2007) LGBT couples in later life: a study in diversity. *Generations*, Fall, 18–23.

Dey, I. (2006) Wearing out the work ethic: population ageing, fertility and work–life balance. *Journal of Social Policy* 35, 671–88.

Dobash, R. P. and Dobash, R. P. (1980) *Violence Against Wives.* Shepton Mallet: Open Books.

Dobash, R. P. and Dobash, R. P. (1992) *Women, Violence and Social Change.* London: Routledge.

Donnison, J. (1977) *Midwives and Medical Men: A History of Interprofessional Rivalry and Womens' Rights.* London: Heinemann.

Donovan, C. (2006) Genetics, fathers and families: exploring the implications of changing the law in favour of identifying sperm donors. *Social & Legal Studies* 15, 494–510.

Doucet, A. (2006) *Do Men Mother? Fathering, Care, and Domestic Responsibility.* Toronto, ON: University of Toronto Press.

Dowling, M. and Brown, G. (2009) Globalisation and international adoption from China. *Child and Family Social Work.* Available online at: www.open. ac.uk/hsc/pers/m.s.dowling/pics/d102232.pdf.

Dromgoole, S. (2009) A view from the marketplace: games now and going forwards. Paper presented at Game Based Learning Conference, London. Available online at www.gamebasedlearning2009.com/proceedings/ presentations/904–presentations/226–seandromgoole-ceo-some-research (accessed 3 August 2010).

Drotner, K., Siggaard Jensen, H. and Schroder, K. C. (2008) Conceptual and relational vagaries of learning and media. In K. Drotner, H. Siggaard Jensen and K. C. Schroder (eds.) *Informal Learning and Digital Media.* Cambridge: Cambridge Scholars Publishing, pp. 1–10.

Drury, B. (1991) Sikh girls and the maintenance of ethnic culture. *New Community* 17, 387–99.

Dube, B. R., Dube, R. and Dube, R. (2005) *Female Infanticide in India: A Feminist Cultural History.* New York: State University of New York Press.

Duncan, S. (2007) What's the problem with teenage parents? And what's the problem with policy? *Critical Social Policy* 27, 307–34.

Duncan, S. and Edwards, R. (1999) *Lone Mothers, Paid Work and Gendered Moral Rationalities*. London: Macmillan.

Duncan, S. and Phillips, M. (2008) New families? Tradition and change in modern relationships. In A. Park, J. Curtice, K. Thomson, M. Phillips, M. Johnson and E. Clert (eds.) *British Social Attitudes, the 24th Report*. London: Sage.

Duncan, S. and Smith, D. (2006) Individualisation versus the geography of 'new' families. *Twenty-First Century Society* 1, 167–89.

Dunn, J. and Deater-Deckard, K. (2001) *Children's Views of their Changing Families*. York: Joseph Rowntree Foundation.

Dunne, G. (1997) *Lesbian Lifestyles: Women's Work and the Politics of Sexuality*. London: Macmillan.

Dunne, G. (1999) A passion for sameness? In E. B. Silva and C. Smart (eds.) *The New Family?* London: Sage, pp. 66–82.

Dunne, G. A. (2000) Opting into motherhood: lesbians blurring the boundaries and transforming the meanings of parenthood and kinship. *Gender and Society* 14, 11–35.

Durham, D. (2007) Empowering youth: making youth citizens in Botswana. In J. Cole and D. Durham, *Generations and Globalisation: Youth, Age and Family in the New World Economy*. Bloomington and Indianapolis: Indiana University Press, pp. 102–32.

Dykstra, P. A. (2006) Off the beaten track: childlessness and social integration in late life. *Research on Aging* 28 (6), 749–67.

Dykstra, P. A. and Hagestad, G. O. (2007) Roads less taken: developing a nuanced view of older adults without children. *Journal of Family Issues* 28 (10), 1275–310.

Edgell, S. (1980) *Middle Class Couples*. London: Allen and Unwin.

Edwards, J. (1999) Explicit connections: ethnographic enquiry in North-West England. In J. Edwards, S. Franklin, E. Hirsch, F. Price and M. Strathern (eds.) *Technologies of Procreation: Kinship in the Age of Assisted Conception*. London: Routledge, pp. 60–85.

Edwards, R., Hadfield, L. and Mauthner, M. (2005) *Children's Understandings of their Sibling Relationships*. London: National Children's Bureau.

Ehrenreich, B. (2002) Maid to order. In B. Ehrenreich and A. R. Hochschild (eds.) (2003) *Global Woman: Nannies, Maids and Sex Workers in the New Economy*. London: Granta Books, pp. 85–103.

Ehrenreich, B. and English, D. (1978) *For Her Own Good: 150 Years of the Experts' Advice to Women*. Garden City, NY: Doubleday Anchor.

Ehrenreich, B. and Hochschild, R. (2003) Introduction. In B. Ehrenreich and A. R. Hochschild (eds.) *Global Woman: Nannies, Maids and Sex Workers in the New Economy*. London: Granta Books, pp. 1–14.

Eichler, M. (1981) The inadequacy of the monolithic model of the family. *Canadian Journal of Sociology* 6, 367–88.

Elias, N. (1998) The civilizing of parents. In J. Goudsblom and S. Mennell (eds.) *The Norbert Elias Reader: A Biographical Selection.* Oxford: Blackwell, pp. 189–211.

Engels, F. (1972 [1884]) *The Origin of the Family, Private Property and the State.* London: Lawrence and Wishart.

English Longitudinal Study on Ageing. Available online at www.ifs.org.uk/elsa.

Equality and Human Rights Commission (2009) *Financial Services Inquiry.* London: Equality and Human Rights Commission.

Ermisch, J. (2000) Personal relationships and marriage expectations: evidence from the 1998 British Household Panel Study. *Working Paper 2000–27,* Institute for Social and Economic Research, University of Essex, Colchester, Essex.

Evans, M. (2011) Engels: materialism and morality. In J. Sayers, M. Evans and N. Redclift (eds.) *Engels Revisited: Feminist Essays.* London: Routledge Revivals, pp. 81–97.

Everett, C. (1991) *The Consequences of Divorce.* New York: Haworth Press.

Fan, C. C. and Li, L. (2002) Marriage and migration in transnational China: a field study of Gaozhu, Western Guangdong. *Environment and Planning A* **34**, 619–38.

Farquhar, M.A. (1999) *Children's Literature in China: From Lu Xun to Mao Zedong.* Armonk, NY: M.E. Sharpe.

Featherstone, B. (2004) *Family Life and Family Support: A Feminist Analysis.* Basingstoke: Palgrave Macmillan.

Featherstone, B. (2010) Writing fathers in but mothers out!!! *Critical Social Policy* **30**, 208–24.

Feinberg, J. (2004) The child's right to an open future. In M. Freeman (ed.) *Children's Rights,* Vol.I. Dartmouth, Aldershot and Burlington, VA: Ashgate, pp. 213–42.

Fennell, G., Phillipson, C. and Evers, H. (1988) *The Sociology of Old Age.* Milton Keynes: Open University Press.

Ferguson, N., Douglas, G., Lowe, N., Murch, M. and Robinson, M. (2004) *Grandparenting in Divorced Families.* Bristol: The Policy Press.

Finch, J. (2007) Displaying families. *Sociology* **41**, 65–81.

Finch, J. and Mason, J. (1993) *Negotiating Family Responsibilities.* London: Routledge.

Finch, J. and Summerfield, P. (1991) Social reconstruction and the emergence of companionate marriage, 1945–1959. In D. Clark (ed.) *Marriage, Domestic Life and Social Change.* London: Routledge, pp. 7–32.

Firestone, S. (1970) *The Dialectics of Sex: The Case for Feminist Revolution.* New York: William Morrow and Co.

Firth, R. (1956) *Two Studies of Kinship in London.* London: Athlone.

Fischer, C. (2011) *Still Connected: Family and Friends in America since 1970.* New York: Russell Sage Foundation.

Fischer, T. (2007) Parental divorce and children's socio-economic success: conditional effects of parental resources prior to divorce, and gender of the child. *Sociology* **41**, 475–95.

Flichy, P. (1995) *Dynamics of Modern Communication: The Shaping and Impact of New Communication Technologies.* London: Sage.

Folgerø, T. (2008) Queer nuclear families? Reproducing and transgressing heteronormativity. *Journal of Homosexuality* **54**, 124–49.

Foucault, M. (1978/2001) Governmentality. In J. D. Faubion (ed.) *Essential Works of Foucault 1954–1984: Power,* Vol. III. London: Penguin, pp. 201–222.

Fox Harding, L. (1999) Family values and Conservative government policy. In G. Jagger and C. Wright (eds.) *Changing Family Values.* London: Routledge, pp. 119–35.

Franklin, A. (1989) Working class privatism: an historical case study of Bedminster, Bristol. *Environment and Planning D: Society and Space* **7**, 93–113.

Franklin, S. (1997) *Embodied Progress: A Cultural Account of Assisted Conception.* London: Routledge.

Franklin, S. and Ragone, H. (1998) Introduction. In S. Franklin and H. Ragone (eds.) *Reproducing Reproduction.* Philadelphia: University of Pennsylvania Press, pp. 1–14.

Franklin, S. and McKinnon, S. (2002) *Relative Values: Reconfiguring Kinship Studies.* Durham, NC and London: Duke University Press.

Frosh, S., Phoenix, A. and Pattman, R. (2002) *Young Masculinities: Understanding Boys in Contemporary Society.* London: Palgrave.

Gabb, J. (2004) Critical differentials: querying the incongruities within research on lesbian parent families. *Sexualities* **7**, 167–82.

Gabb, J. (2008) *Researching Intimacy in Families.* London: Palgrave Macmillan.

Gallo, E. (2008) Unorthodox sisters: gender relations and generational change among Malayali migrants in Italy. In R. Palriwala and P. Uberoi (eds.) *Marriage, Migration and Gender.* New Delhi: Palgrave Macmillan, pp. 180–214.

Gamarnikow, E. (1985) *Gender, Class and Work.* London and New York: Gower Publishing.

Gambles, R., Lewis, S. and Rapaport, R. (2006) *The Myth of Work–Life Balance: The Challenge of our Time for Men, Women and Societies.* Chichester: J. Wiley.

Gamburd, M. R. (2002) *Transnationalism and Sri Lanka's Migrant Housemaids.* New Delhi: Vistaar.

Ganatra, B., Hirve, S. and Rao, V. N. (2001) Sex-selective abortion: evidence from a community-based study in Western India. *Asia-Pacific Journal* **16**, 109–24.

Gartrell, N. and Bos, H. (2010) US National Longitudinal Lesbian Family Study: psychological adjustment of 17-year-old adolescents. *Pediatrics* 126. Available online at www.pediatrics.org/cgi/content/full/126/3/617 (accessed 30 April 2011).

Gartrell, N., Deck, A., Rodas, C., Peyser, H. and Banks, A. (2005) The National Lesbian Family Study: 4. Interviews with the 10-year-old children. *American Journal of Orthopsychiatry* **75**, 518–24.

Gentile, D. A., Lynch, P. J., Linder, J. R. and Walsh, D. A. (2004) The effects of violent video game habits on adolescent hostility, aggressive behaviours, and school performance. *Journal of Adolescence* **27**, 5–22.

George, S. M. (2006) Millions of missing girls: from fetal sexing to high technology sex selection in India. *Prenatal Diagnosis* **26**, 604–9.

Gershuny, J. (2001) *Changing Times*. Oxford: Oxford University Press.

Gershuny, J., Godwin, M. and Jones, S. (1994) The domestic labour revolution: a process of lagged adaptation. In M. Anderson, F. Bechhofer and J. Gershuny (eds.) *The Social and Political Economy of the Household*. Oxford: Oxford University Press, pp. 151–97.

Ghuman, P. S. (1999) *Asian Adolescents in the West*. London: British Psychological Society Books.

Ghuman, P. S. (2003) *Divided Loyalties: South Asian Adolescents in the West*. Cardiff: University of Wales Press.

Giddens, A. (1990) *The Consequences of Modernity*. Cambridge: Polity Press.

Giddens, A. (1991) *Modernity and Self Identity*. Cambridge: Polity Press.

Giddens, A. (1992) *The Transformation of Intimacy: Sexuality, Love and Eroticism in Modern Societies*. Cambridge: Polity Press.

Giddens, A. (1998) *The Third Way: The Renewal of Social Democracy*. Cambridge: Polity Press.

Gillies, V. (2005) Raising the 'meritocracy': parenting and the individualisation of social class. *Sociology* **39**, 836–7.

Gillies, V., Ribbens McCarthy, J. and Holland, J. (2001) *'Pulling Together, Pulling Apart': The Family Lives of Young People*. York: Family Policy Studies Centre / Joseph Rowntree Foundation.

Ginn, J. and Arber, S. (1995) 'Only connect': gender relations and ageing. In S. Arber and J. Ginn (eds.) *Connecting Gender and Ageing: A Sociological Approach*. Buckingham: Open University Press, pp. 1–14.

Glynn, S. (2002) Bengali Muslims: the new East End radicals? *Ethnic and Racial Studies* **25**, 969–88.

Goering, J. and Wienk, R. (eds.) (1997) *Mortgage Lending, Racial Discrimination and Federal Policy*. Brookfield: Ashgate.

Goldberg, A. E. (2010) *Gay and Lesbian Parents and Their Children: Research on the Family Life Cycle*. Washington DC: American Psychological Association.

Golombok, S. and Murray, C. (1999) *Egg and Semen Donation: A Survey of UK Licensed Centres*. Report for the National Gamete Donation Trust. London: City University.

Golombok, S., Perry, B., Burston, A., et al. (2003) Children with lesbian parents: a community study. *Developmental Psychology* **39**, 20–33.

Goodman, B. (1977) *The Lesbian: A Celebration of Difference*. New York: Out & Out Books.

Goodman, C. and Silverstein, M. (2001) Grandmothers who parent their grandchildren: an exploratory study of close relations across three generations. *Journal of Family Issues* **22**, 557–78.

Goulbourne, H. and Chamberlain, M.(eds.) (2001) *Caribbean Families in the TransAtlantic World*. London: Macmillan.

Gray, J. (2002) *Men Are from Mars, Women Are from Venus: A Practical Guide for Improving Communication and Getting What You Want in Your Relationships*. London: Harper Element.

Green, R. (1992) *Sexual Science and the Law*. Cambridge, MA: Harvard University Press.

Greenberg, J. and Muehlebach, A. (2007) The Old world and its new economy: notes on the 'Third Age' in Western Europe today. In J. Cole and D. Durham (eds.) *Generations and Globalization: Youth, Age, and Family in the New World Economy*. Bloomington: Indiana University Press.

Greer, G. (1970) *The Female Eunuch*. London: Paladin.

Grewal, I. and Kishore, J. (2008) Female foeticide in India. *International Humanist and Ethical Union*. Available online at www.iheu.org/node/1049 (accessed 23 August 2011).

Griffith, A. and Smith, D. (2005) *Mothering for Schooling*. London: Routledge Falmer.

Grobstein, C. and Flower, M. (1985) Current ethical issues. *Clinics in Obstetrics and Gynecology* **12**, 887–91.

Gross, N. (2005) The detraditionalisation of intimacy reconsidered. *Sociological Theory* **23**, 286–311.

Guilmoto, C. Z. (2007) Characteristics of sex-ratio imbalance in India and future scenarios. Paper presented at the United Nations Populations Fund Fourth Asia Pacific Conference on Reproductive and Sexual Health Rights. Available online at www.unfpa.org/gender/docs/studies/india.pdf.

Gulati, L. (1993) *In the Absence of their Men: The Impact of Male Migration on Women*. New Delhi: Sage.

Gupta, J. A. (2006) Towards transnational feminisms: some reflections and concerns in relation to the globalization of reproductive technologies. *European Journal of Women's Studies* **13**, 23–38.

Haber, C. and Gratton, B. (1994) *Old Age and the Search for Security: An American Social History*. Bloomington, IN: Indiana University Press.

Haddon, L. (2004) *Information and Communication Technologies in Everyday Life: A Concise Introduction and Research Guide*. Oxford: Berg.

Haddon, L. (2006). Empirical studies using the domestication framework. In T. Berker, M. Hartmann, Y. Punie and K. J. Ward (eds.), *Domestication of Media Technology*. Maidenhead: Open University Press, pp. 103–22

Haimes, E. (1990) Recreating the family? Policy considerations relating to the 'new' reproductive technologies. In M. McNeil, I. Varcoe and S. Yearley (eds.) *The New Reproductive Technologies*. Basingstoke: Macmillan Press, pp. 154–72.

Haimes, E. (1993) Issues of gender in gamete donation. *Social Science and Medicine* 36, 85–93.

Haimes, E. (1998) The making of the 'DI child': changing representations of people conceived through donor insemination. In K. Daniels and E. Haimes (eds.) *Donor Insemination: International Social Science Perspectives*. Cambridge: Cambridge University Press, pp. 53–75.

Hall, R. A. (2002) When is a wife not a wife? Some observations on the immigration experiences of South Asian women in West Yorkshire. *Contemporary Politics* 9 (1), 55–68.

Han, M. and Eades, J. S. (1995) Brides, bachelors and brokers: the marriage market in rural Anhui in an era of economic reform. *Modern Asian Studies* 29 (4), 841–69.

Hansen, K.V. (2004) The asking rules of reciprocity in networks of care for children. *Qualitative Sociology* 27 (4), 421–37.

Hansen, K.V. (2005) *Not-so-nuclear Families: Class, Gender and Networks of Care*. New Jersey: Rutgers University Press.

Hao, L. (2003) Regarding the United States' refusal to contribute to the U.N. Fund for Population Activities. *Population Research* 1 (27), 17–19.

Harden, J. (2007) There's no place like home: the public/private distinction in children's theorizing of risk and safety. *Childhood* 14, 43–59.

Hardill, I. (2002) *Gender, Migration and the Dual Career Household: Invisible Migrants*. London: Routledge.

Harrison, C. (2008) Implacably hostile or appropriately protective? Women managing child contact in the context of domestic violence. *Violence Against Women* 14 (4), 381–405

Hartmann, H. (1976) Capitalism, patriarchy and job segregation by sex. In M. Blaxall and B. Reagan (eds.) *Women and the Workplace: The Implications of Occupational Segregation*. Chicago: University of Chicago Press, pp. 137–79.

Harvey, D. (1989) *The Condition of Postmodernity*. Oxford: Basil Blackwell.

Haskey, J. (1999) Cohabitational and marital histories of adults in Great Britain. *Population Trends* 96, 13–23.

Haskey, J. (2001) Cohabitation in Great Britain: past, present and future trends and attitudes. *Population Trends* **103**, 4–25.

Haskey, J. (2005) Living arrangements in contemporary Britain: having a partner who lives elsewhere and Living Apart Together (LAT). *Population Trends* **122**, 35–45.

Hatmadji, S. H. and Wiyono, N. H. (2008) Support transfers between elderly parents and adult children in Indonesia. In L. Hock Guan (ed.) *Ageing in Southeast and East Asia: Family, Social Protection and Policy Challenges.* Singapore: Institute of Southeast Asian Studies, pp. 230–44.

Hauari, H. and Hollingworth, K. (2009) *Understanding Fathering: Masculinity, Diversity and Change.* York: Joseph Rowntree Foundation. Available online at www.jrf.org.uk/publications/understanding-fathering. (accessed 30 April 2011).

Haub, C. and Sharma, O. P. (2006) India's population reality: reconciling change and tradition. *Population Bulletin* 61 (3), 1–19. Available online at www.globalmedicine.nl/index.php/gm8–november-2009/160–indias-missing-women.

Heaphy, B. (2009) The storied complex lives of older GLBT adults: choice and its limits in older lesbian and gay narratives of relational life. *Journal of GLBT Family Studies* **5**, 119–38.

Heaphy, B., Donovan, C. and Weeks, J. (1999) Sex, money and the kitchen sink: power in the same sex couple relationship. In J. Seymour and P. Bagguley (eds.) *Relating Intimacies: Power and Resistance.* London: Macmillan, pp. 222–45.

Heaphy, B., Yip, A. K. T. and Thompson, D. (2003) *Lesbian, Gay and Bisexual Lives over 50.* Nottingham: York House Publications.

Heaphy, B., Yip, A. K. T. and Thompson, D. (2004) Ageing in a non-heterosexual context. *Ageing and Society* **24**, 881–902.

Heim, J., Bae Brandtzæg, P., Hertzberg Kaare, B., Endestad, T. and Torgersen, L. (2007) Children's usage of media technologies and psychosocial factors. *New Media and Society* **9**, 425–54.

Henwood, K. and Proctor, J. (2003) The 'good father': reading men's accounts of paternal involvement during the transition to first time fatherhood. *British Journal of Social Psychology* **42**, 337–56.

Hertz, R. (2006) *Single by Chance, Mothers by Choice: How Women Are Choosing Parenthood Without Marriage and Creating the New American Family.* Oxford: Oxford University Press.

Hey, V. (1997) *The Company She Keeps: An Ethnography of Girls' Friendships.* Buckingham: Open University Press.

Heycox, K. (1997) Older women: issues of gender. In A. Borowski, S. Encel and E. Ozanne (eds.) *Ageing and Social Policy in Australia.* Melbourne: Cambridge University Press, pp. 94–118.

HFEA (Human Fertilization and Embryology Authority) (2006) *SEED Report:*

A Report on the Human Fertilization and Embryology Authority's Review of Sperm, Egg and Embryo Donation in the United Kingdom. London: HFEA.

Hines, A. (1997) Divorce-related transitions, adolescent development and the role of the parent–child relationship. *Journal of Marriage and Family* **59**, 375–88.

Hobson, B. (2002) (ed.) *Making Men into Fathers: Men, Masculinities and the Social Politics of Fatherhood.* Cambridge: Cambridge University Press.

Hochschild, A. (1983) *The Managed Heart: Commercialization of Human Feeling.* Berkeley: University of California Press.

Hochschild, A. R. (1989) *The Second Shift.* New York: Viking Penguin.

Hochschild, A. R. (1995) The culture of politics: traditional, postmodern, cold-modern, and warm-modern ideas of care. *Social Politics* **2**, 331–46.

Hochschild, A. R. (2000) Global care chains and emotional surplus values. In W. Hutton and A. Giddens (eds.) *On the Edge: Living with Global Capitalism.* London: Jonathan Cape, pp. 130–46.

Hochschild, A. R. (2003a) Love and gold. In B. Ehrenreich and A. R. Hochschild (eds.) *Global Woman: Nannies, Maids and Sex Workers in the New Economy.* London: Granta Books, pp. 15–30.

Hochschild, A. R. (2003b) *The Commercialisation of Intimate Life: Notes from Home and Work.* Berkeley, CA: University of California Press.

Hock Guan, L. (2008) Introduction. In L. Hock Guan (ed.) *Ageing in Southeast and East Asia: Family, Social Protection and Policy Challenges.* Singapore: Institute of Southeast Asian Studies, pp. 1–21.

Hoff, A. and Tesch-Romer, C. (2007) Family relations and aging: substantial changes since the middle of the last century? In H.-W. Wahl, C. Tesch-Romer and A. Hoff (eds.) *New Dynamics in Old Age.* Amityville: Baywood Publishing Co., pp. 65–84.

Hofferth, S. J. and Owens, T. J. (eds.) (2001) *Children at the Millennium: Where Have We Come From, Where Are We Going?* New York: JAI.

Holden, K. (2007) *The Shadow of Marriage: Singleness in England, 1914–1960.* Manchester: Manchester University Press.

Homans, H. (1986) *The Sexual Politics of Reproduction.* Aldershot: Gower.

Horst, H. (2008) Families. In M. Ito, S. Baumer, M. Bittanti et al. (eds.) *Hanging Out, Messing Around, Geeking Out: Living and Learning with New Media.* Cambridge, MA: MIT Press, pp. 123–57.

Houston, D. M. (2005) *Work–Life Balance in the Twenty-First Century.* Basingstoke: Palgrave Macmillan.

Inhorn, M. (2005) Fatwas and ARTS: IVF and gamete donation in Sunni v. Shi'a Islam. *Journal of Gender, Race and Justice* **9**, 291–318.

Inhorn, M. C. (2007) Reproductive disruptions and assisted reproductive technologies. In M. C. Inhorn (ed.) *Reproductive Disruptions: Gender, Technology, and Biopolitics in the New Millennium.* Oxford: Berghahn Books, pp. 183–99.

Iyer, S. (2002) *Demography and Religion in India*. Oxford: Oxford University Press.

Izuhara, M. (2010) Introduction. In M. Izuhara (ed.) *Ageing and Intergenerational Relations: Family Reciprocity from a Global Perspective*. Cambridge: Polity Press, pp. 1–12.

James, A. and Prout, A. (eds.) (1997) *Constructing and Reconstructing Childhood*. 2nd edn. London: Routledge/Falmer.

James, A., Jenks, C. and Prout, A. (1998) *Theorizing Childhood*. Cambridge: Polity Press.

Jamieson, L. (1987) Theories of family development and the experience of being brought up. *Sociology* **21**, 591–607.

Jamieson, L. (1998) *Intimacy: Personal Relationships in Modern Societies*. Cambridge and Malden, MA: Polity Press.

Jamieson, L. (1999) Intimacy transformed: a critical look at the pure relationship. *Sociology* **33**, 477–94.

Jamieson, L., Anderson, M., McCrone, D., Bechhofer, F., Stewart, R. and Li, Y. (2002) Cohabitation and commitment: partnership plans of young men and women. *Sociological Review* **18**, 253–70.

Jayaram, N. (ed.) (2004) *The Indian Diaspora: Dynamics of Migration*. London: Sage.

Jenks, C. (1996) *Childhood*. London: Routledge.

Jha P., Kumar, R., Vasa, P. et al. (2006) Low male-to-female sex ratio of children born in India: national survey of 1.1 million households. *The Lancet* **367** (9506), 211–18.

Johnson, E. (2007) *Dreaming of a Mail-order Husband: Russian–American Internet Romance*. Durham NC: Duke University Press.

Johnson, M. (1990) *Staying Power: Long term Lesbian Couples*. Tallahassee, FL: Naiad Press.

Johnson, S. M. and O'Connor, E. (2002) *The Gay Baby Boom: The Psychology of Gay Parenthood*. New York: New York University Press.

Johnston, R. J., Taylor, P. J. and Watts, M. J. (eds.) (2002) *Geographies of Global Change*. Oxford: Basil Blackwell.

Jones, A. F. (2002) The child as history in Republican China: a discourse on development. *Positions: East Asia Cultures Critique* **10**, 695–727.

Jones, I. R., Leontowitsch, M. and Higgs, P. (2010) The experience of retirement in second modernity: generational habitus among retired senior managers. *Sociology* **44**, 103–20.

Jonsson, J. O. and Gähler, M. (1997) Family dissolution, family reconstitution, and children's educational careers: recent evidence for Sweden. *Demography* **34**, 277–93.

Kahani-Hopkins, V. and Hopkins, N. (2002) 'Representing' British Muslims: the strategic dimension of identity construction. *Ethnic and Racial Studies* **25**, 288–309.

Kakabadase, A. and Kakabadse, N. (2004) *Intimacy: An International Survey of the Sex Lives of People at Work*. Basingstoke: Palgrave Macmillan.

Kalmijn, M. (1994) Mother's occupational status and children's schooling. *American Sociological Review* **59**, 257–75.

Kalpagam, U. (2008) 'American *Varan*' marriages among Tamil Brahmans: preferences, strategies and outcomes. In R. Palriwala and P. Uberoi (eds.) *Marriage, Migration and Gender*. New Delhi: Sage, pp. 98–124.

Kaur, R. (2004) Across-region marriages: poverty, female migration and the sex ratio. *Economic and Political Weekly* **39** (25): 2595–603.

Kehily, M. J. (2010) Childhood in crisis? Tracing the contours of 'crisis' and its impact upon contemporary parenting practices. *Media, Culture & Society* **32**, 171–85.

Keil, T. and Andreescu, V. (1999) Fertility policy in Ceausescu's Romania. *Journal of Family History* **24**, 478–92.

Khanum, S. (2001) The household patterns of a 'Bangladeshi village' in England. *Journal of Ethnic and Migration Studies* **27**, 489–504.

Kiernan, K. (1999) Cohabitation in Western Europe. *Population Trends* **96**, 25–32.

Kiernan, K., Land, H. and Lewis, J. (1998) *Lone Motherhood in Twentieth Century Britain*. Oxford: Oxford University Press.

Kiernan, K. E., Barlow, A. and Merlo, R. (2007) Cohabitation law reform and its impact on marriage: evidence from Australia and Europe. *International Family Law* **63**, 71–4.

King, R. and Vullnetari, J. (2006) Orphan pensioners and migrating grandparents: the impact of mass migration on older people in rural Albania. *Ageing and Society* **26**, 783–816.

King, V., Harris, K. and Heard, H. (2004) Racial and ethnic diversity in nonresident father involvement. *Journal of Marriage and Family* **66**, 1–21.

Kitzinger, S. (1978) *Women as Mothers: How They See Themselves in Different Cultures*. New York: Vintage Books.

Klein, J. (2005) Irregular marriages: unorthodox working-class domestic life in Liverpool, Birmingham, and Manchester 1900–1939. *Journal of Family History* **30**, 210–29.

Kligman, G. (1992) The politics of reproduction in Ceausescu's Romania: a case study in political culture. *East European Politics and Societies* **6**, 364–418.

Kligman, G. (1998) *The Politics of Duplicity: Controlling Reproduction in Ceausescu's Romania*. Berkeley, CA: University of California Press.

Kohli, M., Kundermund, H., Motel, A. and Szydlik, M. (2000) Families apart: intergenerational transfers in East and West Germany. In S. Arber and C. Attias-Donfut (eds.) *The Myth of Generational Conflict: The Family and State in Ageing Societies*. London: Routledge, pp. 88–99.

König, A. (2008) Which clothes suit me? The presentation of the juvenile self. *Childhood* **15**, 225–37.

Konrad, M. (2005) *Nameless Relations: Anonymity, Melanesia and Reproduction. Gift Exchange between British Ova Donors and Recipients*. New York and Oxford: Berghahn Books.

Koser, K. and Lutz, H. (eds.) (1998) *The New Migration in Europe*. London: Macmillan.

Kotchick, B. and Forehand, R. (2002) Putting parenting in perspective: a discussion of the contextual factors that shape parenting practices. *Journal of Child and Family Studies* **11** (3), 255–69.

Kuhn, A. and Wolpe, A. (eds.) (1978) *Feminism and Materialism: Women and Modes of Production*. London: Routledge & Kegan Paul.

Lamb, M. E. (1995) The changing role of fathers. In J. L. Shapiro, M. J. Diamond and M. Geenburg (eds.) *Becoming a Father*. New York: Springer, pp. 18–35.

Lamb, S. (2000) *White Saris and Sweet Mangoes: Aging, Gender and Body in North India*. Berkeley, CA: University of California Press.

Lamb, S. (2007) Aging across worlds: modern seniors in an Indian diaspora. In J. Cole and D. Durham, *Generations and Globalisation: Youth, Age and Family in the New World Economy*. Bloomington and Indianapolis: Indiana University Press, pp. 132–63.

Lan, T.Y. (2003) Population aging in Taiwan: future health implications. *Taiwan Journal of Public Health* **22**, 237–44.

Landale, N. S., Thomas, K. J. A. and Van Hook, J. (2011) The living arrangements of children of immigrants. *Immigrant Children* **21** (1), 43–70.

Lareau, A. (2002) Invisible inequality: social class and childrearing in black and white families. *American Sociological Review* **67**, 747–76.

Lareau, A. (2003) *Unequal Childhoods: Class, Race and Family Life*. Berkeley, CA: University of California Press.

LaRossa, R. (1988) Fatherhood and Social Change. *Family Relations* **37**, 451–7.

Lasch, S. (1979) *The Culture of Narcissism*. London: Abacus.

Laslett, P. (2005 [1965]) *The World We Have Lost – Further Explored*. London: Abacus.

Layard, R. and Dunn, J. (2009) *A Good Childhood: Searching for Values in a Competitive Age*. London: Penguin.

Lehmann, P. and Wirtz, C. (2004) Household formation in the EU – lone parents. *Statistics in Focus* (EUROSTAT, Luxembourg) Special Issue: Population and Social Conditions, Theme 3, 5/2004, 1–8. Available online at http://epp.eurostat.ec.europa.eu/cache/ITY_OFFPUB/KS-NK-04–005/EN/KS-NK-04–005–EN.PDF.

Leonard, D. (1980) *Sex and Generation*. London: Tavistock.

Leonardo, M. (1987) The female world of cards and holidays: women, families, and the work of kinship. *Signs* **12**, 440–53.

Levitt, P. (2001) *The Transnational Villagers*. Berkeley, CA: University of California Press.

Lewis, C. and Lamb, M. E. (2007) *Understanding Fatherhood: A Review of Recent Research*. York: Joseph Rowntree Foundation.

Lewis, J. (1999) *Marriage, Cohabitation and the Law: Individualism and Obligation*. Research Series no. 1/99. London Lord Chancellor's Department.

Lewis, J. (2001) *The End of Marriage: Individualism and Intimate Relations*. Cheltenham: Edward Elgar Publishing.

Lewis, J. and Campbell, M. (2007) UK work–family balance policies and gender equality. *Social Politics* **14**, 4–30.

Lewis, J. with Datta, J. and Sarre, S. (1999) *Individualism and Commitment in Marriage and Cohabitation*. Research Series no. 8/99. London: Lord Chancellor's Department.

Lewis, R. and Smee, S. (2009) Closing the gap: does transparency hold the key to unlocking pay equality? *Gender Equality Forum*. London: Fawcett Society. Available online at www.fawcettsociety.org.uk/documents/Closing%20the%20Gap%20–%20does%20transparency%20hold%20the%20key%20to%20unlocking%20pay%20equality%281%29.pdf (accessed 10 April 2011).

Liang, Q. and Lee, C. (2006) Fertility and population policy: an overview. In D. L. Poston, C. Lee, C. Chang, S. L. McKibben and C. S. Walther (eds.) (2009) *Fertility, Family Planning and Population Policy in China*. London and New York: Routledge, pp. 7–19.

Lincoln, S. (2004) Teenage girls' bedroom culture: codes versus zones. In A. Bennett and K. Harris (eds.) *After Subculture: Critical Studies of Subcultural Theory*. Basingstoke: Palgrave Macmillan, pp. 94–106.

Lister, R. (2006) Children (but not women) first: New Labour, child welfare and gender. *Critical Social Policy* **26**, 315–36.

Lister, R. (2009) A Nordic nirvana? Gender, citizenship and social justice in the Nordic welfare states. *Social Politics* **16**, 242–79.

Liu, C. and Chang, C. (2006) Patterns of sterilization. In D. L. Poston, C. Lee, C. Chang, S. L. McKibben and C. S. Walther (eds.) *Fertility, Family Planning and Population Policy in China*. London and New York: Routledge, pp. 38–50.

Livingstone, S. (2002) *Young People and New Media: Childhood and the Changing Media Environment*. London: Sage.

Livingstone, S. (2009) *Children and the Internet*. Cambridge: Polity Press.

Logan, S. (ed.) (1996) *The Black Family: Strengths, Self-Help, and Positive Change*. Boulder, CO: Westview.

Longino, C. F., Jackson, D. J., Zimmerman, R. S. and Bradsher, J. (1991) The second move: health and geographic mobility. *Journal of Gerontology* **46**, 218–24.

Lowenstein, A. and Daatland, S. O. (2006) Filial norms and family support in a comparative cross-national context: evidence from the OASIS study. *Ageing and Society* **26**, 203–24.

Lu, M. C. (2008) Commercially arranged marriage migration: case studies of cross-border marriages in Taiwan. In R. Palriwala and P. Uberoi (eds.) *Marriage, Migration and Gender*. New Delhi: Sage. pp. 125–51.

Macfarlane, A. (1979) *The Origins of English Individualism: The Family, Property and Social Transition*. Cambridge: Cambridge University Press.

Mackay, H. (1997) Consuming communication technologies at home. In H. Mackay (ed.) *Consumption and Everyday Life*. London: Sage, pp. 259–308.

Maclean, M. (1991) *Surviving Divorce*. Basingstoke: Macmillan.

Macleod, D. I. (1998) *The Age of the Child: Children in America, 1890–1920*. New York: Twayne Publishers.

Maher, J. and Saugeres, L. (2007) To be or not to be a mother? Women negotiating cultural representations of mothering. *Journal of Sociology* **43** (1), 5–21.

Malinowski, B. (1932) *The Sexual Life of Savages in North-Western Melanesia*. 3rd edn. London: Routledge & Kegan Paul.

Mamo, L. (2007) *Queering Reproduction: Achieving Pregnancy in the Age of Technoscience*. Durham, NC: Duke University Press.

Mand, K. (2008) Marriage and migration through the life course: experiences of widowhood, separation and divorce amongst transnational Sikh women. In R. Palriwala and P. Uberoi (eds.) *Marriage, Migration and Gender*. New Delhi: Sage, pp. 286–303.

Mansfield, P. and Collard, J. (1987) *The Beginning of the Rest of Your Life? A Portrait of Newly-Wed Marriage*. London: Macmillan.

Manthorpe, J. (2003) Nearest and dearest? The neglect of lesbians in caring relationships. *British Journal of Social Work* **33**, 753–68.

Manting, D. (1996) The changing meaning of cohabitation and marriage. *European Sociological Review* **121**, 53–65.

Marsh, M. and Ronner, W. (1996) *The Empty Cradle: Infertility in America from Colonial times to the Present*. Baltimore, MD: Johns Hopkins University Press.

Mason, D. (2000) *Race and Ethnicity in Modern Britain*. Oxford: Oxford University Press.

May, E. (1995) *Barren in the Promised Land: Childless Americans and the Pursuit of Happiness*. New York: Basic Books.

May, V. (2001) *Lone Motherhood in Finnish Women's Life Stories*. Abo: Abo Akademi University Press.

May, V. (2003) Lone motherhood past and present: the life stories of Finnish lone mothers. *Nordic Journal of Women's Studies* **11** (1), 27–39.

May, V. (2008) On being a 'good' mother: the moral presentation of self in written life stories. *Sociology* **42**, 470–86.

Mayall, B. (2002) *Towards a Sociology for Childhood: Thinking from Children's Lives*. Buckingham: Open University Press.

McCray, C.A. (1980) The Black woman and family roles. In L. Rodgers-Rose (ed.) *The Black Woman*. Beverley Hills, CA: Sage.

McDowell, J. (2004) *Child Support Handbook*. London: Child Poverty Action.

McKay, D. (2003) Filipinas in Canada: deskilling as a push towards marriage. In N. Piper and M. Roces (eds.) *Wife or Worker: Asian Women and Migration*. Maryland: Rowman and Littlefield, pp. 23–52.

McLanahan, S. (2007) Single mothers, fragile families. In J. Edwards, M. Crain and A. L. Kalleberg (eds.) *Ending Poverty in America: How to Restore the American Dream*. New York: The New Press, pp. 77–87.

McLoyd, V., Cauce, A., Takeuchi, D. and Wilson, L. (2000) Marital processes and parental socialization in families of color: a decade review of research. *Journal of Marriage and the Family* 62 (4), 1070.

Means, R. (2007) The re-medicalisation of later life. In M. Bernard and T. Scharf (eds.) *Critical Perspectives on Ageing Societies*. Bristol: The Policy Press.

Mears, D. P., Hay, C., Gertz, M. and Mancini, C. (2007) Public opinion and the foundation of the juvenile court. *Criminology* 45, 223–58.

Mehta, K. K. and Leng, T. L. (2008) Multigenerational families in Singapore. In L. Hock Guan (ed.) *Ageing in Southeast and East Asia: Family, Social Protection and Policy Challenges*. Singapore: Institute of Southeast Asian Studies, pp. 216–29.

Meirow, D. and Schenker, J. G. (1997) The current status of sperm donation in assisted reproduction technology: ethical and legal considerations. *Journal of Assisted Reproduction and Genetics* 14, 133–8.

Michielin, F., Mulder, C. H. and Zorla, A. (2008) Distance to parents and geographical mobility. *Population, Space and Place* 14, 327–45.

Millar, J. (2001) Work requirements and labour market programmes for lone parents. In J. Millar and K. Rowlingson (eds.) *Lone Parents, Employment and Social Policy Cross-national Comparisons*. Bristol: The Policy Press, pp. 189–210.

Miller, B. D. (1989) Changing patterns of juvenile sex ratios in rural India, 1961–1971. *Economic and Political Weekly* 24 (22), 1229–36.

Miller, T. (2010) *Making Sense of Fatherhood: Gender, Caring and Work*. Cambridge: Cambridge University Press.

Millet, K. (1970) *Sexual Politics*. New York: Doubleday.

Minkler, M. (1999) Intergenerational households headed by grandparents. *Journal of Aging Studies* 13, 199–218.

Mitchell, J. (1975) *Women and Psychoanalysis*. New York: Vintage Books.

Modood, T., Berthoud, R., Lakey, J. et al. (1997) *Ethnic Minorities in Britain: Diversity and Disadvantage*. London: Policy Studies Institute.

Mogey, J. (1956) *Family and Neighbourhood*. London: Oxford University Press.

Momsen, J. H. (1999) *Gender, Migration and Domestic Service*. London: Routledge.

Morgan, D. (1996) *Family Connections: An Introduction to Family Studies*. Cambridge: Polity Press.

Morgan, D. (1999) Gendering the household: some theoretical considerations. In L. Mckie, S. Bowlby and S. Gregory (eds.) *Gender, Power and the Household*. London: Macmillan, pp. 22–40.

Morgan, D. (2011) *Rethinking Family Practices*. London: Palgrave Macmillan.

Morgan, L. H. (1870) *Systems of Consanguinity and Affinity in the Human Family*. Washington DC: Smithsonian Institute

Moynihan, D. P. (1965) *The Negro Family: A Case for National Action*. Washington DC: Government Printing Office.

Mueller, M. and Elder, G. (2003) Family contingencies across the generations: grandparent–grandchild relationships in holistic perspective. *Journal of Marriage and the Family* 65, 404–17.

Murakami, K., Atterton, J. and Gilroy, R. (2008) *Planning for the Ageing Countryside in Britain and Japan: City-Regions and the Mobility of Older People*. Research Report to the Daiwa Anglo-Japanese Foundation. Available online at: www.ncl.ac.uk/cre/publish/researchreports (accessed on 28 April 2011).

Murdoch, L. (2006) *Imagined Orphans: Poor Families, Child Welfare and Contested Citizenship in London*. New Brunswick, NJ and London: Rutgers University Press.

Naftali, O. (2010) Caged golden canaries: childhood, privacy and subjectivity in contemporary urban China. *Childhood* 17, 297–311.

Nagel, C. (2002) Constructing difference and sameness: the politics of assimilation in London's Arab communities. *Ethnic and Racial Studies* 25, 258–87.

Nardi, P. (1999) *Gay Men's Friendships: Invincible Communities*. Chicago: University of Chicago Press.

National Institute of Population and Social Security Research (1998) *The Eleventh National Family Survey: Marriage and Fertility in Japan*. National Institute of Population and Social Security Survey. Tokyo: National Institute of Population and Social Security Research.

Natividad, J. N. (2008) Family and household conditions of the elderly in Southeast Asia: living arrangements as social support. In L. Hock Guan (ed.) *Ageing in Southeast and East Asia: Family, Social Protection and Policy Challenges*. Singapore: Institute of Southeast Asian Studies, pp. 155–67.

Nazroo, J., Bajekal, M., Blane, D. and Grewal, I. (2004) Ethnic inequalities. In C. Hennessy and A. Walker (eds.) *Growing Older: Quality of Life in Old Age*. Maidenhead: Open University Press.

Negro-Vilar, A. (1993) Stress and other environmental factors affecting fertility in men and women: overview. *Environmental Health in Perspectives* **101** (Suppl. 2), 59–64.

Nelson, J. A. (1998) One sphere or two? *American Behavioural Scientist* **41**, 1467–71.

Nelson, M. (2002) The challenge of self-sufficiency: women on welfare redefining independence. *Journal of Contemporary Ethnography* **31** (5), 582–614.

Nelson, M. (2005) *The Social Economy of Single Motherhood: Raising Children in Rural America*. London: Routledge.

Nelson, M. (2010) *Parenting Out of Control: Anxious Parents in Uncertain Times*. New York: New York University Press.

Nikken, P., Jansz, J. and Schouwstra, S. (2007). Parents' interest in video game ratings and content descriptors in relation to game mediation. *European Journal of Communication* **22**, 315–36.

Nobles, W.W. (1974) Africanity: its role in Black families. *The Black Scholars* **5**, 10–17.

Oakley, A. (1972) *Sex, Gender and Society*. Aldershot: Temple Smith/Gower.

Oakley, A. (1974) *The Sociology of Housework*. London: Martin Robertson.

Obama, B. (2008) *Change We Can Believe In: Barack Obama's Plan to Renew America's Promise*. New York: Three Rivers Press.

O'Brien, M. and Shemilt, I. (2003) *Working Fathers: Earning and Caring*. London: Equal Opportunities Commission.

O'Brien, M., Alldred, P. and Jones, D. (1996) Children's constructions of family and kinship. In J. Brannen and B. O'Brien (eds.) *Children in Families: Research and Policy*. London: Falmer Press, pp. 84–100.

O'Donnell, K. (1999) Lesbian and gay families: legal perspectives. In G. Jagger and C. Wright (eds.) *Changing Family Values*. London: Routledge, pp. 77–97.

Ofcom (2009a) *Digital Lifestyles: Parents of Children under 16*. Available online at http://stakeholders.ofcom.org.uk/market-data-research/media-literacy/medlitpub/medlitpubrss/digilifestyles/ (accessed 3 August 2010).

Office for National Statistics (2000) *Conceptions to Women Aged under 18, England and Wales*. Available online at: www.statistics.gov.uk/statbase (accessed 17 April 2011).

Office for National Statistics (2001) *Census*. London: ONS. Available online at www.ons.gov.uk/census/get-data/index.html (accessed 13 December 2011).

Office for National Statistics (2008a) The proportion of marriages ending in divorce. *Population Trends* **Spring** (131). Available online at www.statistics. gov.uk/downloads/theme_population/Population_Trends_131_web.pdf (accessed 17 April 2011).

Office for National Statistics (2008b) Work and family: two-thirds of Mums are in employment. *Labour Force Survey* **Q2**. Available at www.statistics. gov.uk/cci/nugget.asp?id=1655.

Office for National Statistics (2009) State of the nation. *Social Trends* **39**. Available online at www.statistics.gov.uk/downloads/theme_social/ Social_Trends39/Social_Trends_39.pdf (accessed 17 April 2011).

Office for National Statistics (2010) *Social Trends* **40**. Available online at www.statistics.gov.uk/downloads/theme_social/Social-Trends40/ST 40_2010_FINAL.pdf (accessed 17 April 2011).

Ong, A. and Zhang, L. (2008) Introduction: privatizing China: powers of the self, socialism from afar. In L. Zhang and A. Ong (eds.) *Privatizing China: Socialism from Afar*. 2nd edn. Ithaca, NY: Cornell University Press, pp. 1–20.

Organisation for Economic Cooperation and Development (2005) *Spotlight: Economic and Social Effects of Ageing Population in Japan*. Available online at www.oecd.org/document/63/0,3343,en_33873108_ 33873539_35326655_1_1_1_1,00.html

Oswald, R. F. (2000) Family and friendship relationships after young women come out as bisexual or lesbian. *Journal of Homosexuality* **38**, (3), 65–83.

Owen, C., Peart, E. and Barreau, S. (2006) Looking back: experiences of private fostering. In S. Jackson, E. Chase and A. Simon (eds.) *In and After Care: A Positive Perspective*. London: Cornell University Press, pp. 101–14.

Pahl, J. (1989) *Money and Marriage*. New York: St Martin's Press.

Pahl, R. and Spencer, L. (2001) *Rethinking Friendship: Personal Communities and Social Cohesion*. ESRC report. Available at www.esrc.ac.uk/my-esrc/ grants/R000237836/outputs/Read/8b1b0360–c040–4cc0–b3ad-62d4f33a 99c2.

Palriwala, R. (2003) Dowry in contemporary India: an overview. In AIDWA (All India Democratic Women's Association) *The Practice of Dowry Itself Is a Crime, Not Just Its Excesses: A Report on the Workshops on Expanding Dimensions of Dowry*. New Delhi: AIDWA and ISWSD, pp. 11–27.

Palriwala, R. and Uberoi, P. (2008) Exploring the links: gender issues in marriage and migration. In R. Palriwala and P. Uberoi (eds.) *Marriage, Migration and Gender*. New Delhi: Sage, pp. 23–62.

Pande, A. (2008) Commercial surrogate mothering in India: nine months of labor? In K. Kosaka and M. Ogino (eds.) *Quest for Alternative Sociology*. Melbourne: Trans Pacific Press, pp. 71–88.

Pande, A. (2010) Commercial surrogacy in India: manufacturing a perfect mother-worker. *Signs: Journal of Women in Culture and Society* **35**, 969–92.

Parrenas, R. S. (2001) *Servants of Globalization: Women, Migration and Domestic Work*. Stanford, CA: Stanford University Press.

Parrenas, R. S. (2003) The care crisis in the Philippines: children and transnational families in the new global economy. In B. Ehrenreich and A. R. Hochschild (eds.) *Global Woman: Nannies, Maids, and Sex Workers in the New Economy*. London: Granta Books, pp. 39–54.

Parrenas, R. S. (2005) *Children of Global Migration: Transnational Families and Gendered Woes*. Stanford, CA: Stanford University Press.

Parrenas, R. S. (2006) Caring for the Filipino family: how gender differentiates the economic causes of labor migration. In A. Agrawal (ed.) *Migrant Women and Work*. New Delhi: Sage, pp. 95–115.

Parsons, T. (1942) Age and sex in the social structure of the United States. *American Sociological Review* 7 (5) (Oct.), 604–16.

Parsons, T. (1956) The American family: its relations to personality and to the social structure. In T. Parsons and R. F. Bales (1956) *Family Socialisation and Interaction Process*. London: Routledge & Kegan Paul, pp. 13–33.

Parsons, T. (1971) The normal American family. In B. Adams and T. Weirath (eds.) *Readings on the Sociology of the Family*. Chicago: Markham, pp. 53–66.

Parsons, T. and Bales, R. F. (1956) *Family Socialisation and Interaction Process*. London: Routledge & Kegan Paul.

Patchin, J. W. and Hinduja, S. (2010) Trends in online social networking: adolescent use of MySpace over time. *New Media & Society* 12, 197–216.

Peplau, L. A. and Cochran, S. D. (1990) A relationship perspective on homosexuality. In D. P. McWhirter, S. A. Sanders and J. M. Reinisch (eds.) *Homosexuality/Heterosexuality: Concepts of Sexual Orientation*. New York: Oxford University Press, pp. 321–49.

Phillipson, C. (2007) Migration and health care for older people: developing a global perspective. In K. W. Schaie and P. Uhlenberg (eds.) *Social Structures: Demographic Change and the Well-being of Older Persons*. New York: Springer Publishing, pp. 158–69.

Phillipson, C. (2009) Pensions in crisis: aging and inequality in a global age. In L. Rogne, C. Estes, B. Grossman, B. Hollister and E. Solway (eds.) *Social Insurance and Social Justice*. New York: Springer, pp. 319–40.

Phillipson, C. (2010) Globalisation, global ageing and intergenerational change. In M. Izuhara (ed.) *Ageing and Intergenerational Relations*. Bristol. Policy Press, pp. 13–28.

Phillipson, C., Bernard, M., Phillips, J. and Ogg, J. (2001) *The Family and Community Life of Older People*. London: Routledge.

Phillipson, C., Ahmed, N. and Latimer, J. (2003) *Women in Between: A Study of the Experiences of Bangladeshi Women Living in Tower Hamlets*. Bristol: The Policy Press.

Phillipson, C. R., Baars, J., Dannefer, D. and Walker, A.. (2006) *Aging, Globalization and Inequality: The New Critical Gerontology*. New York: Baywood.

Phoenix, A. (1996) Social constructions of lone motherhood: a case of competing discourses. In E. B. Silva (ed.) *Good Enough Mothering?* London: Routledge, pp. 175–90.

Phoenix, A. and Husain, F. (2007) *Parenting and Ethnicity*. York: Joseph Rowntree Foundation.

Plaza, D. (2002) Review of ethnicities: children of immigrants in America. *Journal of Marriage and Family* **64**, 549–56.

Plummer, K. (1995) *Telling Sexual Stories: Power, Change and Social Worlds*. London: Routledge.

Pollack, M. (1979) *Nine Years Old*. London: Heinemann.

Pollock, L. (1983) *Forgotten Children: Parent–Child Relations from 1500 to 1900*. Cambridge: Cambridge University Press.

Poncz, E. (2007) China's proposed International Adoption Law: the likely impact on single U.S. citizens seeking to adopt from China and the available alternatives. *Harvard International Law Journal Online* **48**, 74–82.

Porche, M. and Purvin, D. (2008) 'Never in our lifetime': legal marriage for same-sex couples in long-term relationships. *Family Relations* **57**, 144–59.

Poston, D. L. and Glover, K. S. (2006) China's demographic density: marriage market implications for the twenty-first century. In D. L. Poston Jr, C. Lee, C. Chang, S. L. McKibben and C. S. Walther (eds.) (2009) *Fertility, Family Planning and Population Policy in China*. London and New York: Routledge, pp. 172–86.

Poston, D. L., Jr, Lee, C., Chang, C., McKibben, S. L. and Walther, C. S. (eds.) (2009) *Fertility, Family Planning and Population Policy in China*. London and New York: Routledge.

Prinz, C. (1995) *Cohabiting, Married or Single: Portraying, Analyzing and Modeling New Living Arrangements in the Changing Societies of Europe*. Aldershot: Avebury.

Prout, A. (2002) Researching children as social actors: an introduction to the Children 5–15 Programme. *Children and Society* **16**, 67–79.

Pugh, A. (2009) *Longing and Belonging: Parents, Children and Consumer Culture*. Berkeley, CA: University of California Press.

Purewal, N. K. (2010) *Son Preference: Sex Selection, Gender and Culture in South Asia*. New York: Berg.

Putnam, R. (2000) *Bowling Alone*. New York: Simon and Schuster.

Quilliam, S. (1995) *Relate Guide to Staying Together: From Crisis to Deeper Commitment*. London: Random House.

Qvortrup, J., Bardy, M., Sgritta, G. and Wintersberger, H. (1994) *Childhood Matters: Social Theory, Practice and Politics*. Aldershot: Avebury.

Rainwater, L. and Smeeding, T. M. (2003) *Poor Kids in a Rich Country*. New York: Russell Sage Foundation.

Rake, K. and Lewis, R. (2009) Just below the surface: gender stereotyping, the silent barrier to equality in the modern workplace. *Gender Equality Forum*. London: The Fawcett Society. Available online at www.fawcettsociety.org.uk/documents/JustBelowtheSurface.pdf (accessed 10 April 2011).

Ramanama, A. and Bambawale, U. (1980) The mania for sons: an analysis of social values in South Asia. *Social Science and Medicine* **14B**, 107–10.

Ramesh, R. (2008) India to crack down on doctors aborting girls. *The Guardian*, 25 April 2008, p. 24.

Raymond, J. G. (1993) *Women as Wombs: Reproductive Technologies and the Battle over Women's Freedom*. Melbourne: Spinifex Press.

Reay, D. (1998) *Class Work: Mothers' Involvement in Their Children's Primary Schooling*. London: UCL Press.

Reece, H. (2006) UK women's groups' child contact campaign: 'So long as it is safe'. *Child and Family Law Quarterly* **18** (4), 538–61.

Registrar General (2001) Provisional population totals. *Census of India 2001*. New Delhi: Office of the Registrar General.

Reinier, J. S. (1996) *From Virtue to Character: American Childhood, 1775–1850*. New York: Twayne Publishers.

Reissman, C. K. (2000) Stigma and everyday practices: childless women in South India. *Gender and Society* **14**, 111–35.

Reynolds, T. (2001) Black mothering, paid work and identity. *Ethnic and Racial Studies* **24** (6), 1046–70.

Reynolds, T. (2005) *Caribbean Mothers: Identity and Experience in the UK*. London: Tufnell Press.

Ribbens McCarthy, J. and Edwards, R. (2002) The individual in public and private: the significance of mothers and children. In A. Carling, S. Duncan and R. Edwards (eds.) *Analysing Families: Morality and Rationality in Policy and Practice*. London: Routledge, pp. 199–217.

Ribbens McCarthy, J., Edwards, R. and Gillies, V. (2000) Moral tales of the child and the adult: narratives of contemporary family lives under changing circumstances. *Sociology* **34** (4), 785–803.

Ribbens McCarthy, J., Edwards, R. and Gillies, V. (2003) *Making Families: Moral Tales of Parenting and Step-Parenting*. Durham: Sociology Press.

Rich, A. (1980) Compulsory heterosexuality and lesbian existence. *Signs: Journal of Women in Culture and Society* **5**, 631–60.

Richards, L. (1999) The interests of children at divorce. In G. Allan (ed.) *The Sociology of the Family: A Reader*. Oxford: Blackwell, pp. 262–78.

Riggs, D. W. (2007) *Becoming Parent: Lesbians, Gay Men, and Family*. Teneriffe, Australia: Post Pressed.

Rivers, D. (2010) 'In the best interests of the child': lesbian and gay parenting custody cases, 1967–1985. *Journal of Social History* **Summer**, 917–43.

Robertson, J. (1994) *Children of Choice: Freedom and the New Reproductive Technologies*. Princeton: Princeton University Press.

Robertson, R. (1992) *Globalisation: Social Theory and Global Culture*. London: Sage.

Roche, J. (1999) Children's rights, participation and citizenship. *Childhood* **6**, 475–93.

Rodriguez, G. (2009) Home-based communication system for older adults and their remote family. *Computers in Human Behaviour* **25**, 609–18.

Roschelle, A. R. (1997) *No More Kin: Exploring Race, Class and Gender in Family Networks*. Thousand Oaks, CA: Sage.

Rose, N. (1999) *Governing the Soul: The Shaping of the Private Self*. 2nd edn. London: Routledge.

Rosenbluth, F. M. (ed.) (2007) *The Political Economy of Japan's Low Fertility*. Stanford, CA: Stanford University Press.

Roseneil, S. and Budgeon, S. (2004) Cultures of intimacy and care beyond 'the Family': personal life and social change in the early 21st century. *Current Sociology* **52** (2), 135–59.

Roseneil, S. and Mann, K. (1996) Unpalatable choices and inadequate families: lone mothers and the underclass debate. In E. B. Silva (ed.) *Good Enough Mothering? Feminist Perspectives on Lone Motherhood*. London: Routledge, pp. 191–210.

Rosenfeld, D. (1999) Identity work among lesbian and gay elderly. *Journal of Ageing Studies* **13**, 121–45.

Rosser, C. and Harris, C. C. (1965, 1983) *The Family and Social Change: A Study of Family and Kinship in a South Wales Town*. London: Routledge & Kegan Paul.

Rothman, B. K. (1988) Reproductive technology and the commodification of life. In E. Baruch, A. F. D'Adamo and J. Seager (eds.) *Embryos, Ethics, and Women's Rights: Exploring the New Reproductive Technologies*. New York: Haworth, pp. 95–100.

Rowlingson, K. and McKay, S. (2005) Lone motherhood and socio-economic disadvantage: insights from quantitative and qualitative evidence. *The Sociological Review* **53** (1), 30–49.

Rozario, S. (2005) Singular predicaments: unmarried female migrants and the changing Bangladeshi family. In M. Thapan (ed.) *Transnational Migration and the Politics of Identity*. New Delhi: Sage, pp. 150–80.

Russell, C. (1987) Ageing as a feminist issue. *Women's Studies International Forum* **10** (2), 125–32.

Russell, C. (2007) What do older women and men want? Gender differences in the 'lived experience' of ageing. *Current Sociology* **55**, 173–92.

Ryan-Flood, R. (2009) *Lesbian Motherhood: Gender, Families and Sexual Citizenship*. London: Palgrave.

Saffron, L. (2001) *It's a Family Affair: The Complete Lesbian Parenting Book*. London: Diva Books.

Salway, S., Chowbey, P. and Clarke, L. (2009) *Parenting in Modern Britain: Understanding the Experiences of Asian Fathers*. York: Joseph Rowntree Foundation. Available at www.jrf.org.uk/sites/files/jrf/Asian-fathers-Britain-full.pdf (accessed 1 August 2011).

Samuel, K. (1999) Stress and reproductive failure: an evolutionary approach with applications to premature labor. *American Journal of Obstetrics & Gynaecology* **180**, 272S–274S.

Sargeant, J. (2010) The altruism of pre-adolescent children's perspectives on 'worry' and 'happiness' in Australia and England. *Childhood* **17**, 411–25.

Sassen, S. (2003) Global cities and survival circuits in global woman. In B. Ehrenreich and A. R. Hochschild (eds.) *Global Woman: Nannies, Maids and Sex Workers in the New Economy.* London: Granta Books, pp. 254–74.

Scharf, T., Phillipson, C., Smith, A. and Kingston, P. (2002) *Growing Older in Socially Deprived Areas: Social Exclusion in Later Life.* London. Help the Aged.

Seamark, C. and Lings, P. (2004) Positive experiences of teenage motherhood: a qualitative study. *British Journal of General Practice* **November**, 813–18.

Seery, B. L. and Crowley, M. S. (2000) Women's emotion work in the family: relationship management and the process of building father–child relationships. *Journal of Family Issues* **21** (1), 100–7.

Selman, P. (1996) Teenage motherhood then and now: a comparison of the pattern and outcome of teenage pregnancy in England and Wales in the 1960s and 1980s. In H. Jones and J. Millar (eds.) *The Politics of the Family.* Avebury: Aldershot, pp. 103–28.

Selman, P. (2003) Scapegoating and moral panics: teenage pregnancy in Britain and the United States. In S. Cunningham-Burley and L. Jamieson (eds.) *Families and the State: Changing Relationships.* London: Palgrave Macmillan, pp. 159–86.

Serow, W. J. and Sly, D. (1991) Geographic mobility of the elderly in industrialized societies. In W. Lutz (ed.) *Future Demographic Trends in Europe and North America: What Can We Assume Today?* San Diego, CA: Academic Press, pp. 399–419.

Sharma, B. R., Gupta, N. and Rellhan, N. (2007) Misuse of prenatal diagnostic technology for sex-selected abortions and its consequences in India. *Public Health* **121**, 854–60.

Shavit, Y. and Blossfeld, H. P. (1993) *Persistent Inequality: Changing Educational Attainment in Thirteen Countries.* Boulder, CO: Westview Press.

Shaw, A. (2000) *Kinship and Continuity: Pakistani Families in Britain.* Amsterdam: Harwood.

Sheel, R. (2008) Marriage, money and gender: a case study of the migrant Indian community in Canada. In R. Palriwala and P. Uberoi (eds.) *Marriage, Migration and Gender.* New Delhi: Sage, pp. 215–34.

Shipman, B. and Smart, C. (2007) 'It's made a huge difference': recognition, rights and the personal significance of civil partnership. *Sociological Research Online* **22** (1). Available online at www.socresonline.org.uk/12/1/shipman.html (accessed July 2009).

Shirahase, S. (2007) Women's economic status and fertility: Japan in cross-national perspective. In F. M. Rosenbluth (ed.) *The Political Economy of Japan's Low Fertility*. Stanford, CA: Stanford University Press, pp. 36–59.

Silverstone, R. (2006). Domesticating domestication: reflections on the life of a concept. In T. Berker, M. Hartmann, Y. Punie and K. J. Ward (eds.) *The Domestication of Media Technology*. Maidenhead: Open University Press, pp. 229–48.

Silverstone, R. and Haddon, L. (1996) Design and the domestication of information and communication technologies: technical change and everyday life. In R. Silverstone and R. Mansell (eds.) *Communication by Design: The Politics of Information and Communication Technologies*. Oxford: Oxford University Press, pp. 44–74.

Simpson, B. (1998) *Changing Families*. Oxford: Berg.

Singh, K. (2008) Child custody cases in the context of international migration. In R. Palriwala and P. Uberoi (eds.) *Marriage, Migration and Gender*. New Delhi: Sage, pp. 348–53.

Sinha-Kerkhoff, K. (2005) From India to an Indian diaspora to a Mauritian diaspora: back-linking as means for women to feel good locally. In M. Thapan (ed.) *Transnational Migration and the Politics of Identity*. New Delhi: Sage, pp. 63–98.

Skeggs, B. (2004) *Class, Self and Culture*. London: Routledge.

Small, M. (2002) Achieving community justice through faith-based groups. *Behavioral Sciences and the Law* **20**, (4), 411–22.

Smart, C. (1987) Law and the problem of paternity. In M. Stanworth (ed.) *Reproductive Technologies: Gender, Motherhood and Medicine*. Cambridge: Polity Press, pp. 98–117.

Smart, C. (1999) The 'new parenthood': fathers and mothers after divorce. In E. B. Silva and C. Smart (eds.) *The New Family?* Cambridge: Polity Press, pp. 100–14.

Smart, C. (2004) Retheorising families. *Sociology* **38**, 1043–8.

Smart, C. (2007) *Personal Life*. Cambridge: Polity Press.

Smart, C. and Neale, B. (1999) *Family Fragments?* Cambridge: Polity Press.

Smart. C. and Shipman, B. (2004) Visions in monochrome: marriage and the individualisation thesis. *Sociology* **55**, 491–509.

Smart, C. and Stevens, P. (2000) *Cohabitation Breakdown*. London: Family Policy Studies Centre / Joseph Rowntree Foundation.

Smith, A., Lalonde, R. N. and Johnson, S. (2004) Serial migration and its implications: a retrospective analysis of the children of Caribbean immigrants. *Cultural Diversity and Ethnic Minority Psychology* **10**, 107–22.

Social Exclusion Unit (SEU) (1999) *Teenage Pregnancy*. Cm 4342. London: HMSO.

Soule, A., Babb, P., Evandrou, M., Balchin, S. and Zealey, L. (2005) *Focus on*

Older People. Basingstoke: Office for National Statistics / Department for Work and Pensions / Palgrave Macmillan.

Spencer, L. and Pahl. R. (2006) *Rethinking Friendship: Hidden Solidarities Today*. Princeton, NJ: Princeton University Press.

Srinivas, M. N. (1984) *Some Reflections on Dowry*. New Delhi: Oxford University Press.

Stacey, J. (1994) The new family values crusaders: Dan Quayle's revenge. *The Nation* **259**, 119–22.

Stacey, J. (1999) Virtual social science and the politics of family values in the United States. In G. Jagger and C. Wright (eds.) *Changing Family Values*. London: Routledge, pp. 185–205.

Stacey, J. and Biblarz, T. J. (2001). (How) does the sexual orientation of parents matter? *American Sociological Review* **66**, 159–83.

Stanley, L. and Wise, S. (1983) *Breaking Out*. London: Routledge.

Stanworth, M. (ed.) (1987) *Reproductive Technologies: Gender, Motherhood and Medicine*. Cambridge: Polity Press

Staples, R. and Mirande, A. (1980) Racial and cultural variations among American families: a decennial review of the literature of minority families. *Journal of Marriage and the Family* **42**, 157–73.

Strasbourg,V. C. and Wilson, B. J. (2002) *Children, Adolescents and the Media*. London: Sage.

Strathern, M. (1992) The meaning of assisted kinship. In M. Stacey (ed.) *Changing Human Reproduction: Social Science Perspectives*. London: Sage, pp. 119–47.

Strathern, M. (2005) *Kinship, Law and the Unexpected*. Cambridge: Cambridge University Press.

Subrahmanyam, K. and Greenfield, P. (2008). Online communication and adolescent relationships. *Project Muse* **18**, 119–46.

Sullivan, O. (2000) The division of domestic labour: twenty years of change? *Sociology* **34**, 437–56.

Taylor, B. (2005) Whose baby is it? The impact of reproductive technologies on kinship. *Human Fertility* **8**, 189–95.

Taylor, P. J.,Watts, M. and Johnston, R. J. (2002) Geography/globalisation. In R. J. Johnston, P. J. Taylor and M. Watts (eds.) *Geographies of Global Change: Remapping the World*. 2nd edition. Malden, MA: Blackwell, pp. 1–17.

Taylor, Y. (2007) *Working-class Lesbian Life: Classed Outsiders*. Basingstoke: Palgrave Macmillan.

Therborn, G. (2004) *Between Sex and Power: Family in the World 1900–2000*. London: Routledge.

Thompson, C. (2005) *Making Parents: The Ontological Choreography of Reproductive Technologies*. Cambridge, MA: The MIT Press.

Thompson, E., Jr (ed.) (1994) *Older Men's Lives*. Thousand Oaks, CA: Sage.

Tienda, M. and Haskins, R. (2011) Immigrant children: introducing the issue. *Immigrant Children* **21** (1), 3–18.

Toliver, S. (1998) *Black Families in Corporate America*. Thousand Oaks, CA: Sage.

Tonnies, F. (1955 [1887]) *Community and Association*. London: Routledge & Kegan Paul.

Torres, S. (2006) Culture, migration, inequality and 'periphery' in a globalized world: challenges for ethno-and anthropogerontology. In J. Baars, D. Dannefer, C. Phillipson and A. Walker (eds.) *Aging, Globalization and Inequality: The New Critical Gerontology*. Amityville: Baywood Publishing Company, pp. 231–44.

Townsend, N. W. (2002). *The Package Deal: Marriage, Work and Fatherhood in Men's Lives*. Philadelphia: Temple University Press.

Townsend, P. (1957) *The Family Life of Old People*. Penguin: Harmondsworth.

Ulicsak, M. and Cranmer, S. (2010) *Gaming in Families: Final Report*. Bristol: Futurelab, Innovation in Education. Available online at www.future lab.org.uk/resources/documents/project_reports/Games_Families_Final _Report.pdf (accessed 11 July 2010).

Ulicsak, M., Wright, M. and Cranmer, S. (2009) *Gaming in Families: A Literature Review*. Bristol: Futurelab, Innovation in Education. Available online at www.futurelab.org.uk/resources/publications-reports-articles/ literature-reviews/Literature-Review1377 (accessed 11 July 2010).

UNICEF (2003) *Teenage Births in Rich Nations*. Innocenti Report Card 3. Florence: UNICEF Innocenti Research Centre.

UNICEF (2007) *Child Poverty in Perspective: An Overview of Child Well-being in Rich Countries*. Innocenti Report Card 7. Florence: UNICEF Innocenti Research Centre.

United Nations (1989) *Convention on the Rights of the Child*. Office of the United Nations High Commissioner for Human Rights. Available online at www2.ohchr.org/english/law/pdf/crc.pdf (accessed on 28 April 2011).

United Nations Population Fund (1999) *The State of the World Population 1999*. Press summary, Information and External Relations Division. Available online at www.unfpa.org/swp/1999/pdf/summary.pdf (accessed 15 April 2011).

United States Bureau of Labor Statistics (2010a) Labor force participation rates among mothers. Available at www.bls.gov/opub/ted/2010/ ted_20100507_data.htm.

United States Census Bureau (2010b) *Marriage and Divorce*. Available at www.census.gov/hhes/socdemo/marriage/data/acs/index.html.

Van Balen, F. and Inhorn, M. C. (2002) Introduction: interpreting infertility – a view from the social sciences. In M. C. Inhorn and F. van Balen (eds.) *Infertility Around the Globe: New Thinking on Childlessness, Gender and*

Reproductive Technologies. Berkeley, CA: University of California Press, pp. 3–32.

Vandebosch, H. and Van Cleemput, K. (2009) Cyberbullying among youngsters: profiles of bullies and victims. *New Media & Society* 11, 1349–71.

Van Every, J. (1999) From modern nuclear family households to postmodern diversity? The sociological construction of families. In G. Jagger and C. Wright (eds.) *Changing Family Values*. London: Routledge, pp. 165–84.

Vann, R. T. (1982) The youth of centuries of childhood. *History and Theory* 21, 279–97.

Van Rompaey, V., and Roe, K. (2001). The home as a multimedia environment: families' conception of space and the introduction of information and communication technologies in the home. *Communications* 26, 351–69.

Van Rooij, F., van Balen, F. and Hermanns, J. M. A. (2004) A review of Islamic Middle Eastern migrants: traditional and religious cultural beliefs about procreation in the context of infertility treatment. *Journal of Reproductive and Infant Psychology* 22, 321–31.

Victor, C., Scrambler, S., Bond, J. and Bowling, A. (2004) Loneliness in later life: preliminary findings from the Growing Older Project. In A. Walker and C. Hennessey (eds.) *Quality of Life in Old Age*. Maidenhead: Open University Press, pp 107–26.

Vincent, C. (1996) *Parents and Teachers: Power and Participation*. London: Falmer Press.

Vincent, C. and Ball, S. (2006) *Childcare, Choice and Class Practices: Middle-Class Parents and their Children*. London: Routledge.

Vincent, C. and Ball, S. (2007) 'Making up' the middle-class child: families, activities and class dispositions. *Sociology* 41, 1061–77.

Vincent, C., Ball, S. J. and Kemp, S. (2004) The social geography of childcare: making up a middle-class child. *British Journal of Sociology of Education* 25, 229–44.

Vuori, J. (2001) *Mothers, Fathers and Professionals: Gender, Repetition and Variety in Expert Texts*. Tampere, Finland: Tampere University Press.

Walby, S. (1985) *Patriarchy at Work*. Cambridge: Polity Press.

Walker, A. and Walker, C. (eds.) (1997) *Britain Divided*. London: Child Poverty Action Group.

Wall, R. (1998) Intergenerational relationships past and present. In A.Walker (ed.) *The New Generational Contract: Intergenerational Relationships, Old Age and Welfare.*, London: UCL Press, pp. 37–55.

Wallach, G. (1997) *Obedient Sons: The Discourse of Youth and Generations in American Culture 1630–1860*. Amherst: University of Massachusetts Press.

Wallbank, J (2007) Getting tough on mothers: regulating contact and residence. *Feminist Legal Studies* 15 (2), 189–222.

Wallerstein, J. S. and Kelly, J. B. (1980) *Surviving the Breakup: How Children and Parents cope with Divorce*. London: Grant McIntyre.

Warin, J., Solomon,Y., Lewis, C. and Langford, W. (1999) *Fathers, Work and Family Life*. London: Family Policy Studies Centre / Joseph Rowntree Foundation.

Warner, M. (1991) Introduction: fear of a Queer planet. *Social Text* **9** (4 [29]), 3–17.

Warnock, M. (1985) *A Question of Life: The Warnock Report on Human Fertilisation and Embryology*. Oxford: Basil Blackwell.

Weeks, J. (1985) *Sexuality and its Discontents: Meanings, Myths and Modern Sexualities*. London: Routledge & Kegan Paul.

Weeks, J. (1995) *Invented Moralities: Sexual Values in an Age of Uncertainty*. Cambridge: Polity Press.

Weeks, J., Heaphy, B. and Donovan, C. (1999a) Everyday experiments: narratives of non-heterosexual relationships. In E. Silva and C. Smart (eds.) *The 'New' Family?* London: Sage, pp. 83–99.

Weeks, J., Heaphy, B. and Donovan, C. (1999b) Partnership rites: commitment and ritual in non-heterosexual relationships. In J. Seymour and P. Bagguley (eds.) *Relating Intimacies: Power and Resistance*. Basingstoke: Macmillan, pp. 43–63.

Weeks, J., Heaphy, B. and Donovan, C. (2001) *Same Sex Intimacies: Families of Choice and Other Life Experiments*. London: Routledge.

Wellman, B. (1979) The community question. *American Journal of Sociology* **84**, 1201–31.

Wells, K. (2009) *Childhood in a Global Perspective*. Cambridge: Polity Press.

Westermarck, E. (1921) *History of Human Marriage*. London: Macmillan and Co.

Weston, K. (1991) *Families We Choose: Lesbians, Gays, Kinship*. New York: Columbia University Press

Weston, K. (2001) *Kinship Controversy*. New York: Columbia University Press.

Widge, A. (2005) Seeking conception: experiences of urban Indian women with in vitro fertilisation. *Patient Education and Counselling* **59**, 226–33.

Williams, C. (2006) *Inside Toyland*. Berkeley, CA: University of California Press.

Williams, F. (2004) *Rethinking Families*. London: Calouste Gulbenkian Foundation.

Williams, S. (2008) What is fatherhood? Searching for the reflexive father. *Sociology* **42**, 487–502.

Willmott, P. (1963) *The Evolution of a Community*. London: Routledge & Kegan Paul.

Willmott, P. and Young, M. (1960) *Family and Class in a London Suburb*. London: Routledge & Kegan Paul.

Wilson, H. and Huntington, A. (2005) Deviant mothers: the construction of teenage motherhood in contemporary discourse. *Journal of Social Policy* **35**, 59–76.

Wilson, W. J. (1991) Studying inner-city social dislocations: the challenges of public agenda research, 1990 Presidential Address. *American Sociological Review* **56**, 1–14.

Winterton, A. (1989) *Impregnation of Lesbian Women*. Early Day Motion 1324. London: House of Commons.

Woodroffe, J. (2009) *Not Having It All: How Motherhood Reduces Women's Pay and Employment Prospects*. London: The Fawcett Society. www.fawcettsociety.org.uk/documents/NotHavingItAll.pdf (accessed 10 April 2011).

Woronov, T. E. (2007) Chinese children, American education: globalizing childrearing in contemporary China. In J. Cole and D. Durham (eds.) *Generations and Globalization: Youth, Age, and Family in the New World Economy*. Bloomington, IN: Indiana University Press, pp. 29–51.

Wright, C. and Jagger, G. (1999) End of century, end of family? Shifting discourse of family crisis. In G. Jagger and C. Wright (eds.) *Changing Family Values*. London: Routledge, pp. 17–37.

Wrigley, J. (1989) Do young children need intellectual stimulation? Experts' advice to parents 1900–1985. *History of Education* **29**, 41–75.

Wu, J. and Walther, C. (2006) Patterns of induced abortion. In D. L. Poston Jr, C. Lee, C. Chang, S. L. McKibben and C. S. Walther (eds.) *Fertility, Family Planning and Population Policy in China*. London and New York: Routledge, pp. 23–33.

Yip, A. (2004) Negotiating space with family and kin in identity construction: the narratives of British non-heterosexual Muslims. *Sociological Review* **52** (3), 336–50.

Young, E., Seale, C. and Bury, M. (1998) 'It's not like family going is it?' Negotiating friendship towards the end of life. *Mortality* **3**, 27–42.

Young, M. and Willmott, P. (1957, 1987) *Family and Kinship in East London*. London: Routledge & Kegan Paul.

Zelizer, V. A. (1985) *Pricing the Priceless Child: The Changing Social Value of Children*. New York: Basic Books.

Zelizer, V. A. (2005) *The Purchase of Intimacy*. Princeton, NJ: Princeton University Press.

Zimmerman, C. C. (1947) *Family and Civilization*. New York: Harper.

Zlotnik, H. (2003) The global dimensions of female migration. *Migration Information Source* (MPI, Washington, DC).

Index